# Impulsivity
## and
# Compulsivity

# Impulsivity
# and
# Compulsivity

**Edited by**

**John M. Oldham, M.D.**
**Eric Hollander, M.D.**
**Andrew E. Skodol, M.D.**

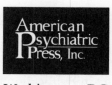

Washington, DC
London, England

Copyright © 1996 American Psychiatric Press, Inc.
ALL RIGHTS RESERVED
Manufactured in the United States of America on acid-free paper
99   98   97   96      4   3   2   1

American Psychiatric Press, Inc.
1400 K Street, N.W., Washington, DC   20005

**Library of Congress Cataloging-in-Publication Data**
Impulsivity and compulsivity  /   edited by John M. Oldham,
   Eric Hollander, and Andrew E. Skodol
         p.         cm.
   Includes bibliographical references and index.
   ISBN 0-88048-676-7 (alk. paper)
   1. Impulsive personality. 2. Compulsive behavior. I. Oldham,
John M. II. Hollander, Eric, 1957–     . III. Skodol, Andrew E.
   [DNLM: 1. Compulsive Behavior. 2. Impulsive Behavior.
3. Obsessive-Compulsive Disorder.     WM 176 I34 1996]
   RC569.5.I46I48 1996
   616.85′2—dc20
   DNLM/DLC
   for Library of Congress                                         95-46597
                                                                        CIP

**British Library Cataloguing in Publication Data**
A CIP record is available from the British Library.

# Contents

# Contributors

**Robert Cloninger, M.D.**
Wallace Renard Professor, Department of Psychiatry, Washington University, St. Louis, Missouri

**Emil F. Coccaro, M.D.**
Professor of Psychiatry, Medical College of Pennsylvania and Hahnemann University, Philadelphia, Pennsylvania

**Lisa J. Cohen, Ph.D.**
Assistant Professor of Psychiatry, Mt. Sinai School of Medicine, New York, New York; Director, Outpatient Specialty Programs, Mt. Sinai Services/Queens Hospital Center, Jamaica, New York

**Eric Hollander, M.D.**
Professor of Psychiatry and Director, Clinical Psychopharmacology and Compulsive, Impulsive and Anxiety Disorders Program, Mt. Sinai School of Medicine, New York, New York

**Richard J. Kavoussi, M.D.**
Associate Professor of Psychiatry, Medical College of Pennsylvania and Hahnemann University, Philadelphia, Pennsylvania

**John M. Oldham, M.D.**
Director, New York State Psychiatric Institute; Chief Medical Officer, New York State Office of Mental Health; Professor of Clinical Psychiatry and Associate Chairman, Department of Psychiatry, Columbia University College of Physicians and Surgeons, New York, New York

**J. Christopher Perry, M.P.H., M.D.**
Professor of Psychiatry and Director of Research, McGill
University at the Institute of Community & Family Psychiatry,
Sir Mortimer B. Davis–Jewish General Hospital, Montreal,
Quebec, Canada; Harvard Medical School at the Austen Riggs
Center, Stockbridge, Massachusetts

**Leon Salzman, M.D.**
Clinical Professor of Psychiatry, Georgetown University School
of Medicine, Washington, D.C.; Past President, American
Academy of Psychoanalysis

**Larry J. Siever, M.D.**
Professor of Psychiatry, Mt. Sinai School of Medicine, New York,
New York; Director of Ambulatory Services, Bronx VA Medical
Center, Bronx, New York

**Andrew E. Skodol, M.D.**
Professor of Clinical Psychiatry, Columbia University College of
Physicians and Surgeons; Director, Unit for Personality Studies,
New York State Psychiatric Institute, New York, New York

**Dan J. Stein, M.B.**
Director of Research, Department of Psychiatry, University of
Stellenbosch, Tygerberg, South Africa

**Michael H. Stone, M.D.**
Professor of Clinical Psychiatry, Columbia University College of
Physicians and Surgeons, New York, New York

**Susan C. Vaughan, M.D.**
Instructor in Clinical Psychiatry, Columbia University College of
Physicians and Surgeons; Candidate, Columbia Center for
Psychoanalytic Training and Research, New York, New York

**Elizabeth Weinberg, M.D.**
Assistant Professor of Psychiatry, Baylor College of Medicine;
Attending Psychiatrist, Quentin Mease Hospital, Houston, Texas

**Mary C. Zanarini, Ed.D.**
Director, Laboratory for the Study of Adult Development,
McLean Hospital, Belmont, Massachusetts; Assistant Professor
of Psychology, Harvard Medical School, Boston, Massachusetts

# Introduction

Traditionally, psychopathological states characterized by impulsive behavior, such as substance abuse, rage outbursts, violence, suicidal or self-destructive acts, binge eating, sexual promiscuity, or social irresponsibility, have been conceptualized as disorders of deficient impulse control. These behaviors have been thought to be fundamentally distinct from, if not diametric to, the phenomena of disorders of *over*control such as obsessional thinking or compulsive behavior.

Patients, however, often present with admixtures of impulsive and compulsive behavior. The clinical criteria used to define disorders as essentially impulsive or compulsive in nature are not always convincing that the fundamental *essence* of the disorder is impulsive or compulsive. DSM-IV[1] classifies a group of disorders as "impulse-control disorders not elsewhere classified"; these disorders are intermittent explosive disorder, kleptomania, pyromania, pathological gambling, trichotillomania, and impulse-control disorder not otherwise specified. DSM-IV also refers to other disorders that "may have features that involve problems of impulse control" (p. 609), including substance-related disorders, paraphilias, antisocial personality disorder, conduct disorder, schizophrenia, and mood disorders. (Most researchers would also include borderline personality disorder on this list.) Although DSM-IV does not similarly specify disorders characterized by compulsivity, the disorders usually included in such a grouping are

---

[1] American Psychiatric Association: *Diagnostic and Statistical Manual of Mental Disorders*, 4th Edition. Washington, D.C., American Psychiatric Association, 1994.

obsessive-compulsive disorder, body dysmorphic disorder, hypochondriasis, depersonalization disorder, anorexia nervosa, Tourette's disorder, and obsessive-compulsive personality disorder.

As defined by DSM-IV, the "essential feature" of impulse-
control disorders is "the failure to resist an impulse, drive, or temptation to perform an act that is harmful to the person or to others"
(p. 609). Yet the criteria for many of these disorders include both
impulsive behavior and behavior seemingly designed to regiment
and control behavior (i.e., to keep impulsive episodes from hap-
pening). For example, what is most central about pathological
gambling—impulsivity or compulsivity? Although pathological
gambling is classified as an impulse-control disorder, the diagnostic criteria for this disorder include one criterion—"is preoccupied
with gambling (e.g., preoccupied with reliving past gambling experiences, handicapping or planning the next venture, or thinking of ways to get money with which to gamble)"—that seems
closer to repetitive obsessional thinking than to deficient impulse
control.

Similarly, some comorbidity studies have found significant co-
occurrences in the same patients of disorders presumably at different ends of the impulsivity-compulsivity spectrum, such as
borderline personality disorder and obsessive-compulsive personality disorder,[2] a counterintuitive combination. To some extent,
these complexities may be more apparent than real, a by-product
of our traditional reliance on descriptive classification. Yet DSM-IV
cautions that

> there is no assumption that each category of mental disorder
> is a completely discrete entity with absolute boundaries divid-
> ing it from other mental disorders or from no mental disorder.
> There is also no assumption that all individuals described as
> having the same mental disorder are alike in all important
> ways. The clinician using DSM-IV should therefore consider

---

[2] Oldham JM, Skodol AE, Kellman HD, et al.: "Diagnosis of DSM-III-R Personality Disorders: Patterns of Comorbidity by Two Structured Interviews." *American
Journal of Psychiatry* 149:213–220, 1992.

that individuals sharing a diagnosis are likely to be heterogeneous even in regard to the defining features of the diagnosis and that boundary cases will be difficult to diagnose in
any but a probabilistic fashion. (p. xxii)

Notwithstanding the usefulness of a descriptive approach to psychopathology, the limitations of such an approach need to be recognized, and the dynamic interaction of (sometimes contradictory)
biopsychosocial forces must be considered as well.

Increasingly, interest in a spectrum model of psychopathology
is developing—in this case, a spectrum of abnormal behavior ranging from impulsivity at one extreme to compulsivity at the other.
Implicit in such a model is the assumption that underlying biological factors determine in part a given patient's degree of impulsivity and/or compulsivity. The serotonergic system has been
studied extensively, with accumulating evidence that low serotonergic system activity is associated with impulsive behavior[3] and
high serotonergic system activity is associated with compulsive
behavior.[4] Other neurotransmitters are inevitably at work in
combination with the serotonergic system, and this, along with
the important contributions of developmental life events in
shaping disordered behavior, adds to the complexity and diversity of behavior.

In this volume, we include contributions from researchers and
clinicians who are active and experienced in this field, to survey
this concept of an impulsivity-compulsivity spectrum. We attempt
to approach the subject from phenomenological, biological, psychodynamic, and treatment perspectives. In the concluding chapter, Dr. Siever provides a brief recapitulation of the ideas presented in each chapter, followed by a synthesis of these ideas, to

---

[3] Kavoussi RJ, Coccaro EF: "Impulsive Personality Disorders and Disorders of
Impulse Control," in *Obsessive-Compulsive–Related Disorders*. Edited by Hollander
E. Washington, D.C., American Psychiatric Press, 1993, pp 179–202.

[4] Hollander E, Fay M, Cohen B, et al.: "Serotonergic and Noradrenergic Sensitivity in Obsessive-Compulsive Disorder: Behavioral Findings." *American Journal
of Psychiatry* 145:1015–1017, 1988.

propose a unified, dynamic way of thinking about impulsive and compulsive behavior.

John M. Oldham, M.D.
Eric Hollander, M.D.
Andrew E. Skodol, M.D.

# 1

## Phenomenology, Differential Diagnosis, and Comorbidity of the Impulsive-Compulsive Spectrum of Disorders

Andrew E. Skodol, M.D.
John M. Oldham, M.D.

Despite the predominance of a categorical approach to the diagnosis of mental disorders, as exemplified by official classifications such as DSM-IV (American Psychiatric Association 1994) and ICD-10 (World Health Organization 1992), interest in spectrum models of psychopathology is increasing. Although psychiatric diagnostic categories resonate with medical tradition in presumptively labeling disease entities with specific etiologies and in facilitating communication and decision making, they also often appear to crudely and imprecisely "carve [human] nature at its joints" (Woods 1979, p. 912). One hypothetical dimension of psychopathology of current interest is the spectrum of impulsive and compulsive thought and behavior. In this chapter we discuss the clinical features of disorders believed to lie on this spectrum, present guidelines for their differential diagnosis, and identify common patterns of codiagnosis or comorbidity.

# Emergence of Interest in Spectra of Psychopathology

Emerging discontent with simplistic categorical models of mental disorders arises from several converging lines of reasoning. Despite rigorous attempts to define homogeneous categories in DSM-III (American Psychiatric Association 1980), DSM-III-R (American Psychiatric Association 1987), and DSM-IV, many of these categories remain heterogeneous. Furthermore, variation within diagnostic categories has been found to have important clinical and research implications. In addition, specific types of cognitions, emotions, behaviors, and interpersonal styles can be observed to cut across many different diagnostic categories. Also, the more rigorous the assessment (e.g., in research studies employing structured diagnostic interviews), the more evident it becomes that many patients have symptoms that meet the criteria for multiple disorders, both on Axis I and Axis II. Thus, "comorbidity" has become the rule in psychiatric diagnosis (Skodol 1989).

In expanding beyond the boundaries of major mental illnesses such as schizophrenia and the mood disorders, psychobiological research has led to the discovery of abnormalities in specific neurotransmitter functions in a wide variety of disparately classified disorders. Family studies have demonstrated familial aggregation of disorders of apparently different types. Treatment studies have indicated that pharmacological agents, such as antidepressant drugs, can benefit patients with many seemingly distinctive types of psychopathology.

Thus, the notion that all 200+ DSM-IV categories represent discrete disorders with distinctive etiologies and pathogenetic mechanisms is patently naive, and the search is on for more fundamental psychopathological disturbances. Groups of clinically observed disorders might be found to cluster together in predictable ways, and each might be a manifestation of one or more basic, underlying disturbances interacting with environmental influences, such as negative life events, chronic adverse circumstances, or cultural factors, to produce psychopathology. Individual disorders, in this model, might differ according to gender or on nondiscrete variables such as severity, duration, stage or phase of illness or of life, aspect(s) of functioning affected, or underlying personality or temperament.

A theory postulating a spectrum of impulsive and compulsive disorders has been gaining momentum primarily because of growing research on abnormalities in serotonin function and experience in treating patients with selective serotonin reuptake inhibitors. These developments are discussed later in this volume.

Impulsive and compulsive behaviors may, at first, seem to be polar opposites on a continuum of control, both control of the self and control of others. Impulsive behaviors seem to be characterized by inadequate or deficient control, resulting in behavioral disinhibition; compulsive behaviors seem to be characterized by excessive overcontrol and behavioral inhibition. Such a simplistic division, however, does not appear to apply when the phenomenology of so-called impulsive and compulsive behaviors is examined more closely. Similarities in the manifestations of illness in both impulsive and compulsive types of disorders lend further support to the existence of a shared continuum of psychopathology.

Cerebral dysfunction clearly contributes to the etiology of some disturbances in the impulsive-compulsive spectrum; in other disturbances, central nervous system (CNS) dysfunction is implicated, if not documented. These disturbances are commonly referred to as "neuropsychiatric." Even for these conditions, however, the etiology of the behavioral disturbance is most often multifactorial and involves neurological, characterological, social, and situational factors. Most of the disorders considered in this chapter have no definitively known etiologies.

## Impulsive and Compulsive Manifestations of Neuropsychiatric Disorders

The first consideration in the differential diagnosis of impulsive or compulsive behaviors is to rule out neuropsychiatric disturbances. Epilepsy, frontal lobe syndromes, hypothalamic-limbic syndromes, metabolic disturbances, substance intoxications and withdrawal states, and psychotic disorders due to general medical conditions are associated with incidences of impulsive, often violent behaviors (Cummings 1985; Fogel and Stone 1992). Other, "nonorganic" disorders such as attention-deficit/ hyperactivity disorder (ADHD) and Tourette's disorder should also be considered as potential causes of certain types of impulsivity. Mental retardation, autism, Lesch-Nyhan syndrome, and choreoacanthocytosis are often associated with self-injurious impulsivity. Obsessive thoughts and/or compulsive behaviors may be seen in association with Parkinson's disease and parkinsonism due to other causes, levodopa therapy in parkinsonism, amphetamine intoxication, frontotemporal CNS trauma or neoplasm, vascular incidents, epilepsy, complex partial seizures, dementias, autism, Klüver-Bucy syndrome, and Tourette's disorder (Cummings 1985).

> A 71-year-old married woman suffered a small stroke in the temporoparietal region of the CNS. In addition to having problems with dysarthria and gait as a result of the stroke, she found herself "compelled" to perform certain repetitive behaviors. In particular, she was touching objects in the household, including lamps and faucets, and checking to make sure closet and medicine cabinet doors were closed and electric stove controls were turned off. She repeatedly wiped off the kitchen sink with a sponge, dried it, and then wiped it with the sponge again. She was preoccupied with making sure her venetian blinds were all slanted in the same direction. Periods of touching, checking, cleaning, or arranging could persist for several hours. If she did not give in to the urge to perform these activities, she felt quite anxious. Before the stroke, she claims to have been "very casual" about housekeeping.

Medical history (including birth and developmental histories), physical (including neurological) examination, mental status examination, and basic laboratory testing of blood and urine may suggest a neurological or other general medical condition as an etiologic factor in the occurrence of impulsive or compulsive behavior (Ovsiew 1992). Neuropsychological testing, electroencephalogram, computed tomography scan, and magnetic resonance imaging may also be indicated for differential diagnosis.

The symptoms of ADHD in adults (e.g., hot temper, affective lability, impulsivity [Wender et al. 1981]) often blend into some of the impulsive behaviors of patients with personality disorders (see discussion later in chapter). ADHD is four to nine times more frequent in males than in females (American Psychiatric Association 1994), and only a minority (about 10%) of children with ADHD (uncomplicated by conduct disorder) have symptoms that persist into adulthood (Mannuzza et al. 1993). Adults who are diagnosed with ADHD should, by definition, have had the full syndrome as children (with the onset of symptoms and impairment before age 7 years). Personality disorders may have childhood antecedents (e.g., conduct disorder), however, making a definitive differential diagnosis difficult.

The verbal outbursts and motor tics of Tourette's disorder, although impulsive in the sense of representing loss of control, have certain compulsive features (see discussion later in chapter). Tics are, however, typically less complex behaviors than are compulsions and are not aimed at reducing anxiety associated with an obsession. Conscious awareness of somatosensory urges and the more complex motor tics of Tourette's disorder can be very difficult to distinguish from obsessions and compulsions (Leckman 1993), and between 30% and 90% of patients with Tourette's disorder also receive a diagnosis of obsessive-compulsive disorder (OCD) (Cummings 1985). Tourette's disorder is more common in males than in females.

A 12-year-old boy was brought to the clinic by his mother, who was becoming increasingly intolerant of her son's "habits." Since age 4, the patient had recurrent periods of facial grimacing and eye twitching, which took the form, alternatively, of a forced smile, bilateral eyebrow raising, or exaggerated blinking. Just before coming to the clinic, he developed a "spitting" habit and a slightly audible, muffled "bark." Family history was positive in that the patient's father had "nervous mannerisms," including a facial tic and grimace. The boy stated that his tics became more frequent whenever he saw or heard his parents arguing. He had great difficulty resisting the tics, even though he knew they annoyed his parents.

## Impulsivity and Compulsivity Associated With Major Mental Disorders

Various behavioral manifestations of impulsivity or compulsivity are also seen in association with major mental disorders, such as schizophrenia, major depressive disorder, and bipolar disorder (American Psychiatric Association 1994). In particular, patients with schizophrenia often engage in impulsive behaviors, including substance abuse, suicide attempts, and acts of violence toward others. Some behavioral disturbances observed in schizophrenia—for example, pacing, rocking, or other stereotyped movements—have driven, compulsive qualities. During major depressive episodes, patients are often prone to suicidal acts and substance use, which reflect deficits in impulse control. Depressed patients also often obsessively ruminate about mood-congruent themes (e.g., having a serious disease or being a terrible or worthless person). In manic episodes, patients typically indulge in impulsive behaviors without concern for the potential consequences of these behaviors. Manic patients may go on unrestrained buying sprees, have indiscriminate sexual encounters, make foolish business investments, gamble excessively, commit unethical acts, or be physically assaultive or self-destructive.

In some instances, impulsive and compulsive behaviors are appropriately viewed as essential or associated features of a psychotic or mood disorder and do not require an additional diagnosis. In other cases, when certain types of behaviors, such as substance use, are particularly severe or maladaptive or require clinical attention or treatment in their own right, additional, comorbid diagnoses from the impulsive-compulsive spectrum of disorders will apply (see discussion later in chapter).

# Core Disorders in the Impulsive-Compulsive Spectrum

Once neuropsychiatric and other major mental disorders are ruled out as causes of impulsivity or compulsivity, the "core" disorders of the impulsive-compulsive spectrum remain. Disorders that are candidates for the spectrum are traditionally labeled impulsive or compulsive. Impulsive disorders are usually thought to include substance use disorders, paraphilias, bulimia nervosa, and impulse-control disorders not elsewhere classified on Axis I and borderline and antisocial personality disorders on Axis II. Compulsive disorders are usually thought to include OCD, body dysmorphic disorder, hypochondriasis, anorexia nervosa, and trichotillomania on Axis I and obsessive-compulsive personality disorder on Axis II. Other disorders possibly occupying places in the spectrum are depersonalization disorder and certain psychotic disorders.

## Axis I Impulsive Disorders

### Substance Use Disorders

Substance use disorders have traditionally been considered manifestations of poor impulse control. Criteria for substance abuse and dependence include items referring to behaviors such as taking more of a substance than intended; trying repeatedly and unsuccessfully to cut down on use; using substances when expected to perform some role obligation or when it is physically hazardous; and using substances despite knowing that they are causing social, psychological, or physical problems. All of these behaviors certainly strongly suggest poor control over the impulse to use substances.

It is interesting, however, that the changes in the concept of *psychoactive substance dependence* in DSM-III-R, away from the purely physiological manifestations of tolerance and withdrawal (as in DSM-III), were meant to introduce an element many addiction specialists believed to be missing from the dependence concept in DSM-III. The revised definition emphasized the "compulsive nature of drug taking or impaired control over drug use" (Skodol 1989, p. 133). Thus, with respect to psychoactive substance use disorders, compulsivity in behavior might be viewed as a loss of behavioral control, or, conversely, poor impulse control might be reflected in behaviors being compulsively performed.

In DSM-IV, the emphasis on the "pattern of compulsive substance use that is characteristic of [d]ependence" (American Psychiatric Association 1994, p. 178) that was introduced by DSM-III-R is perpetuated. (The diagnostic criteria for substance dependence in DSM-III-R and DSM-IV are presented for comparison in Table 1–1.) Items 3 through 7 describe the compulsive drug-taking behavior, and because only three items need to be present for a diagnosis of dependence, "neither tolerance nor withdrawal is necessary or sufficient." According to DSM-IV, individuals with cannabis dependence, for example, often show a pattern of compulsive use without any signs of tolerance or withdrawal.

In DSM-III-R, *substance abuse* was a residual category for diagnosing "maladaptive patterns of psychoactive substance use that have never met the criteria for dependence for that particular class of substance" (American Psychiatric Association 1987, p. 169). The criteria for abuse in DSM-IV are broader in that they include substance use resulting in failure to fulfill major role obligations, which was part of the diagnostic criteria for dependence in DSM-III-R, and in recurrent legal problems. Both DSM-III-R and DSM-IV include dependence and abuse categories for the following classes of substances: alcohol, amphetamines or related substances, cannabis, cocaine, hallucinogens, inhalants, opioids, phencyclidine or related substances, and sedatives, hypnotics, or anxiolytics. Both systems have categories of nicotine dependence but not abuse, because nicotine does not cause a clinically significant intoxication state.

**Table 1–1.**  DSM-III-R and DSM-IV diagnostic criteria for substance dependence: a comparison

| DSM-III-R diagnostic criteria for psychoactive substance dependence | DSM-IV diagnostic criteria for substance dependence |
|---|---|
| A.  At least three of the following: | A maladaptive pattern of substance use, leading to clinically significant impairment or distress, as manifested by three (or more) of the following, occurring at any time in the same 12-month period: |
| (1) substance often taken in larger amounts or over a longer period than the person intended | (1) tolerance, as defined by either of the following: |
| (2) persistent desire or one or more unsuccessful efforts to cut down or control substance use | (a) a need for markedly increased amounts of the substance to achieve intoxication or desired effect |
| (3) a great deal of time spent in activities necessary to get the substance (e.g., theft), taking the substance (e.g., chain smoking), or recovering from its effects | (b) markedly diminished effect with continued use of the same amount of the substance |
| (4) frequent intoxication or withdrawal symptoms when expected to fulfill major role obligations at work, school, or home (e.g., does not go to work because hung over, goes to school or work "high," intoxicated while taking care of his or her children), or when substance use is physically hazardous (e.g., drives when intoxicated) | (2) withdrawal, as manifested by either of the following: |
| | (a) the characteristic withdrawal syndrome for the substance (refer to Criteria A and B of the criteria sets for Withdrawal from the specific substances) |
| (5) important social, occupational, or recreational activities given up or reduced because of substance use | (b) the same (or a closely related) substance is taken to relieve or avoid withdrawal symptoms |
| | (3) the substance is often taken in larger amounts or over a longer period than was intended |

*(continued)*

**Table 1–1.** DSM-III-R and DSM-IV diagnostic criteria for substance dependence: a comparison *(continued)*

| DSM-III-R diagnostic criteria for psychoactive substance dependence | DSM-IV diagnostic criteria for substance dependence |
|---|---|
| (6) continued substance use despite knowledge of having a persistent or recurrent social, psychological, or physical problem that is caused or exacerbated by the use of the substance (e.g., keeps using heroin despite family arguments about it, cocaine-induced depression, or having an ulcer made worse by drinking) | (4) there is a persistent desire or unsuccessful efforts to cut down or control substance use |
| (7) marked tolerance: need for markedly increased amounts of the substance (i.e., at least a 50% increase) in order to achieve intoxication or desired effect, or markedly diminished effect with continued use of the same amount | (5) a great deal of time is spent in activities necessary to obtain the substance (e.g., visiting multiple doctors or driving long distances), use the substance (e.g., chain-smoking), or recover from its effects |
| **Note:** The following items may not apply to cannabis, hallucinogens, or phencyclidine (PCP): | (6) important social, occupational, or recreational activities are given up or reduced because of substance use |
| (8) characteristic withdrawal symptoms (see specific withdrawal syndromes under psychoactive substance–induced organic mental disorders [American Psychiatric Association 1987]) | (7) the substance use is continued despite knowledge of having a persistent or recurrent physical or psychological problem that is likely to have been caused or exacerbated by the substance (e.g., current cocaine use despite recognition of cocaine-induced depression, or continued drinking despite recognition that an ulcer was made worse by alcohol consumption) |
| (9) substance often taken to relieve or avoid withdrawal symptoms | *Specify* if: |
| | **With physiological dependence:** evidence of tolerance or withdrawal (i.e., either Item 1 or 2 is present) |
| | **Without physiological dependence:** no evidence of tolerance or withdrawal (i.e., neither Item 1 nor 2 is present) |

B. Some symptoms of the disturbance have persisted for at least 1 month, or have occurred repeatedly over a longer period of time.

## Criteria for severity of psychoactive substance dependence

**Mild:** Few, if any, symptoms in excess of those required to make the diagnosis, and the symptoms result in no more than mild impairment in occupational functioning or in usual social activities or relationships with others.

**Moderate:** Symptoms or functional impairment between "mild" and "severe."

**Severe:** Many symptoms in excess of those required to make the diagnosis, and the symptoms markedly interfere with occupational functioning or with usual social activities or relationships with others. (Because of the availability of cigarettes and other nicotine-containing substances and the absence of a clinically significant nicotine intoxication syndrome, impairment in occupational or social functioning is not necessary for a rating of severe nicotine dependence.)

**In partial remission:** During the past 6 months, some use of the substance and some symptoms of dependence.

**In full remission:** During the past 6 months, either no use of the substance, or use of the substance and no symptoms of dependence.

*Course specifiers* (see American Psychiatric Association 1994 text for definitions):
    Early full remission
    Early partial remission
    Sustained full remission
    Sustained partial remission
    On agonist therapy
    In a controlled environment

*Source.*   American Psychiatric Association: *Diagnostic and Statistical Manual of Mental Disorders*, 3rd Edition, Revised. Washington, DC, American Psychiatric Association, 1987. American Psychiatric Association: *Diagnostic and Statistical Manual of Mental Disorders*, 4th Edition. Washington, D.C., American Psychiatric Association, 1994. Copyright 1987, 1994, American Psychiatric Association. Used with permission.

Substance use disorders share phenomenology with impulse-control disorders not elsewhere classified in DSM-III-R and DSM-IV (see discussion later in chapter). In DSM-IV, substance use disorders are referred to as impulse-control disorders but are not actually required to meet the general criteria for these disorders. Substance abuse and dependence are more prevalent in males than females, as are intermittent explosive disorder, pathological gambling, and pyromania (McElroy et al. 1992). In their inability to control their consumption of food or contain certain sexual appetites, patients with bulimia and paraphilias share behavior dyscontrol in relation to an appetitive drive with patients with substance use disorders. Colloquially, such patients have been referred to as "food addicts" or "sex addicts." Substance abuse is also one of several manifestations of impulsivity that is potentially self-damaging in borderline personality disorder. Substance use disorders have a broad range of ages at onset, with the majority of cases beginning between the teens and the 40s.

In studies, substance use disorders have been found to co-occur frequently with intermittent explosive disorder, pyromania, kleptomania, pathological gambling, trichotillomania, bulimia, and borderline and antisocial personality disorders (McElroy et al. 1992). Given the considerable overlap among these disorders, the question may be not *which* of the impulse-control disorders a patient might have, but rather *how many*—that is, diagnostic complexity is a function of the multiplicity of different impulse-control disturbances that are manifest in any given patient.

**Paraphilias**

Paraphilias are deviant sexual behaviors characterized by "recurrent, intense sexually arousing fantasies, sexual urges, or behaviors" (American Psychiatric Association 1994, p. 522) involving nonhuman objects, the suffering or humiliation of oneself or one's partner, or children or other nonconsenting partners. Although nearly 50 specific paraphilias have been identified (Money 1986), DSM-III-R and DSM-IV include formal criteria for only 8 of the most frequent: exhibitionism, fetishism, frotteurism, pedophilia, sexual masochism, sexual sadism, transvestic fetishism, and voyeurism. The DSM-III-R/DSM-IV paraphilias and the objects or behaviors that are involved in sexual arousal are listed in Table 1–2.

Persons with paraphilias experience intense urges to perform certain sexual acts, which they feel compelled to perform in order to relieve the urges. Most persons with paraphilias describe a release of tension after the act. Thus, paraphilias have some of the characteristic manifestations of impulse-control disorders. Paraphilias are most commonly seen in men, at least in treatment settings. Age at onset typically ranges from adolescence to early adulthood. Patients often have multiple paraphilias; when one paraphilia is treated or subsides, another may emerge or become more prominent (Abel et al. 1988). When, however, does an intense urge to perform an act cease being an impulse and instead become a compulsion? The typical distinction drawn between a paraphilia (or other mental disorders that might colloquially be called "compulsive" [e.g., pathological gambling or alcohol dependence]) and a classic compulsion is that in the former the person derives pleasure from the sexual behavior, whereas in the latter the person experiences distress while performing the behavior and, as in, for example, the case of many persons with OCD, recognizes the senselessness of the behavior. Furthermore, resistance of the paraphilic compulsion is motivated only by the secondary deleterious consequences of the behavior (e.g., if the person encounters legal problems or finds himself or herself repeatedly exposed to sexually transmitted diseases).

A broader consideration of paraphilic behavior places it in a group of so-called compulsive sexual behaviors that include sexual obsessions and sexual compulsions involving more conventional sexual behaviors taken to the extreme. Sexual obsessions are persistent, intrusive sexual thoughts or fantasies that are usually distressing to the patient (Anthony and Hollander 1993). The patient may also engage in some ritualistic behavior, such as frequent church attendance or praying, designed to neutralize the troubling thoughts. Sexual obsessions are therefore more or less typical of the obsessions seen in OCD. Sexual compulsions may involve pro-

**Table 1–2.**    DSM-III-R/DSM-IV paraphilias

| Category | Object or behavior that is sexually arousing |
|---|---|
| Pedophilia | Child or children age 13 years or younger |
| Exhibitionism | Exposure of genitals to unsuspecting stranger |
| Sexual sadism | Real (not simulated) psychological or physical suffering (including humiliation) of a victim |
| Sexual masochism | The act (real, not simulated) of being humiliated, beaten, bound, or otherwise made to suffer |
| Voyeurism | Observing an unsuspecting person who is naked, in the process of disrobing, or engaging in sexual activity |
| Fetishism | Nonliving objects other than female clothing used in cross-dressing or objects designed for sexual stimulation (e.g., vibrator) |
| Transvestic fetishism | Cross-dressing |
| Frotteurism | Touching and rubbing against a nonconsenting person |
| Paraphilia NOS | Feces (coprophilia)<br>Corpse (necrophilia)<br>Lewdness (telephone scatologia)<br>Exclusive focus on part of the body (partialism)<br>Animals (zoophilia)<br>Enemas (klismaphilia)<br>Urine (urophilia) |

*Note.*   NOS = not otherwise specified.
*Source.*   Adapted from Skodol AE: *Problems in Differential Diagnosis: From DSM-III to DSM-III-R in Clinical Practice.* Washington, D.C., American Psychiatric Press, 1989, p. 481. Copyright 1989, American Psychiatric Press. Used with permission.

miscuous behavior, compulsive autoeroticism, or excessive need for sex from a partner in a relationship. Compulsive sexual behavior is thought to be driven more by anxiety reduction mechanisms than by sexual desire (Coleman 1992). Severe excesses of more normative sexual behaviors may become problematic if they are extremely time consuming, cause problems in relationships, or expose the individual to acquired immunodeficiency syndrome (AIDS) or other sexually transmitted diseases.

More men than women appear to have nonparaphilic as well as paraphilic compulsive sexual behaviors (Weissberg and Levay 1986). One clinical study of comorbidity in self-proclaimed "sex addicts" revealed a substantial prevalence of substance dependence and of eating disorders (Sprenkle 1987). Generalized anxiety may serve as an impetus for compulsive sexual behavior as it may for substance use disorders or other addictions (Qualand 1985). Chronic mild depression, or even episodes of severe major depression, may develop as a consequence of compulsive sexual behaviors. Narcissistic, dependent, schizoid (in the case of auto-eroticism), and borderline personality disorders are also thought to be common in patients with nonparaphilic compulsive sexual behaviors (Coleman 1992).

## Bulimia Nervosa

The eating disorder bulimia nervosa can be considered a disorder of impulse control. The diagnostic criteria include items describing recurrent eating binges, a feeling of lack of control over eating behavior, and frequent ingestion of laxatives or self-induced vomiting to prevent weight gain. Bulimia nervosa, however, is characterized also by certain behaviors with obsessive or compulsive elements. Overconcern with body shape and weight might be described as an "obsession." Strict dieting, fasting, or exercise often indicates a high degree of behavioral control.

> A 30-year-old secretary was admitted to a psychiatric hospital for bulimia and depression with suicidal ideation. The patient, who, as a child, had been obese, began binge eating and purging with laxatives during her junior year in high school. Over the years, her weight had fluctuated from 120 to 220 pounds. Most recently, she had been binge eating once or twice daily on high-carbohydrate foods, such as breads, muffins, Graham crackers, and bagels and in the previous 2 months had gained 40 pounds. She was preoccupied with her physical attractive-

ness and spent considerable time examining her body in a full-length mirror, both naked and in multiple outfits with which she tried to make herself appear thinner. Desperate to lose weight, she had escalated her laxative abuse up to 15 tablets per day and had begun to induce vomiting with syrup of ipecac. The patient described her urge to binge as "powerful and irresistible" and felt that she was completely "helpless" in the face of it. Although she found the act of eating somewhat pleasurable and comforting, immediately afterward she was consumed by guilt over her eating and by self-loathing at her overweight appearance. As her eating and purging spiraled out of control, she became increasingly depressed and began to entertain the idea that she would better off dead than forever doomed to repeat her behaviors and remain fat.

Bulimia nervosa occurs much more often in women than in men. The disorder usually begins in adolescence or early adult life. The consuming aspect of bulimic behavior, as in substance abuse, gambling, or sexual excess, is at least initially pleasurable. The compulsive elements in weight control measures are hardly senseless but instead are performed with deliberate purpose. Thus, bulimia nervosa may be, in the final analysis, closer to an impulsive than a compulsive disorder.

Bulimia nervosa has been shown to co-occur with substance use disorders (Herzog et al. 1992; Katz 1992) and the impulse-control disorders kleptomania (McElroy et al. 1991) and trichotillomania (Christenson et al. 1991), both of which also occur more often in women than in men. Bulimia nervosa has also been demonstrated to co-occur significantly with borderline personality disorder (Herzog et al. 1992; Skodol et al. 1993), a disorder that is again more common among women.

### Impulse-Control Disorders Not Elsewhere Classified

Although grouped in a class of disorders that implies a residual category in DSM-III-R and DSM-IV, the impulse-control disorders not elsewhere classified are the prototypic Axis I disorders of impulse control. The essential features are 1) failure to resist an impulse, drive, or temptation to perform some act that is harmful to the person or to others; 2) an increasing sense of tension or arousal before committing the act; and 3) an experience of pleasure, gratification, or relief at the time of committing the act. The following are members of this class of disorders: intermittent explosive disorder, kleptomania, pyromania, pathological gambling, and trichotillomania.

Intermittent explosive disorder may be the purest example of a disorder characterized by loss of control over an impulse—in this case, the aggressive impulse. As several investigators have pointed out (McElroy et al. 1992), however, intermittent explosive disorder as defined in DSM-III-R did not necessarily fit the general criteria for an impulse-control disorder. The four other disorders are characterized by an increasing sense of tension, which again may reflect an urge compelling the person to act, and a sense of pleasure, gratification, or relief on committing the act. The aggressive acts of intermittent explosive disorder may or may not be preceded by a rising sense of tension; after the act, remorse or guilt is more common than pleasure or relief. Pathological gambling was redefined in DSM-III-R by criteria exactly parallel to those of psychoactive substance dependence in order to emphasize the compulsive nature of the gambling. Some of these features remain in the DSM-IV criteria (Table 1–3). Thus, the impulse-control disorders not elsewhere classified may vary in the degree to which their pathognomonic behaviors are spontaneously impulsive versus compellingly compulsive.

Of the impulse-control disorders not elsewhere classified, kleptomania and trichotillomania are more common in clinical samples among women than men; intermittent explosive disorder, pyromania, and pathological gambling have increased prevalence among men. The onset of kleptomania, pyromania, and trichotillomania is usually in childhood. Pathological gambling usually begins in adolescence in males and later in life in females. Intermittent explosive disorder most commonly begins in the period between late adolescence and the third decade.

Studies of patients with impulse-control disorders not elsewhere classified reveal high rates of lifetime comorbidity with other

---

**Table 1–3.**    DSM-IV diagnostic criteria for pathological gambling

A.  Persistent and recurrent maladaptive gambling behavior as
    indicated by five (or more) of the following:

  (1)  is preoccupied with gambling (e.g., preoccupied with reliving
       past gambling experiences, handicapping or planning the
       next venture, or thinking of ways to get money with which to
       gamble)

  (2)  needs to gamble with increasing amounts of money in order
       to achieve the desired excitement

  (3)  has repeated unsuccessful efforts to control, cut back, or stop
       gambling

  (4)  is restless or irritable when attempting to cut down or stop
       gambling

  (5)  gambles as a way of escaping from problems or of relieving
       a dysphoric mood (e.g., feelings of helplessness, guilt, anxiety,
       depression)

  (6)  after losing money gambling, often returns another day to get
       even ("chasing" one's losses)

  (7)  lies to family members, therapist, or others to conceal the
       extent of involvement with gambling

  (8)  has committed illegal acts such as forgery, fraud, theft, or
       embezzlement to finance gambling

  (9)  has jeopardized or lost a significant relationship, job, or
       educational or career opportunity because of gambling

  (10) relies on others to provide money to relieve a desperate
       financial situation caused by gambling

B.  The gambling behavior is not better accounted for by a manic
    episode.

---

*Source.*    American Psychiatric Association: *Diagnostic and Statistical Manual of
Mental Disorders,* 4th Edition. Washington, D.C., American Psychiatric
Association, 1994. Copyright 1994, American Psychiatric Association. Used
with permission.

impulse-control disorders (most commonly, substance use disorders and eating disorders) and with mental disorders of a nonimpulsive nature (most commonly, mood and anxiety disorders).
Specifically, subjects with intermittent explosive disorder almost
always have substance use disorders, and there may be a relation-

ship with ADHD and with personality disorders, as well. In a study of patients with kleptomania, McElroy and co-workers (1991) found that 100% had a mood disorder, 80% had an anxiety disorder (45% OCD), 60% had an eating disorder (60% bulimia), and 50% had a substance use disorder. In pathological gambling, the results of three studies indicated that 83% of patients had a mood disorder, 42% had a substance use disorder, and 22% had an anxiety disorder (most often OCD) (Linden et al. 1986; Ramirez et al. 1983; Roy et al. 1988). In two studies of patients with trichotillomania (Christenson et al. 1991; Swedo et al. 1989), 72% had a mood disorder, 53% had anxiety disorders, and 23% had histories of alcohol or drug abuse. In pyromania, there may also be high rates of substance use, mood disorders, and personality disorders (McElroy et al. 1992).

## Axis I Compulsive Disorders

### Obsessive-Compulsive Disorder

Obsessive-compulsive disorder is prototypic of the compulsive end of the impulsive-compulsive spectrum of disorders. Obsessions are defined in DSM-IV as "persistent ideas, thoughts, impulses, or images that are experienced as intrusive and inappropriate and that cause marked anxiety or distress." Further, "the individual with obsessions usually attempts to ignore or suppress such thoughts or impulses or to neutralize them with some other thought or action" (American Psychiatric Association 1994, p. 418). Compulsions are "repetitive behaviors . . . or mental acts the goal of which is to prevent or reduce anxiety or distress, not to provide pleasure or gratification." It is further pointed out that "in most cases, the person feels driven to perform the compulsion to reduce the distress that accompanies an obsession or to prevent some dreaded event or situation" (American Psychiatric Association 1994, p. 418). Although at first OCD may look like a disorder of overcontrol, a repetitively performed behavior may represent an instance of motor disinhibition and a recurrent, intrusive thought may be a result of disinhibition or loss of control in the cognitive domain. OCD is classified as an anxiety disorder because obsessions are anxiety-provoking and compulsions are anxiety-reducing (Hollander 1993).

> A 19-year-old college student was referred to a psychiatrist by his family doctor. The student had been suffering for close to 10 years from intrusive thoughts that interfered with his ability to concentrate. His first obsession was that he was going to become another boy, who lived on his street in a house that was an exact duplicate of his own. Because he liked himself and knew he was smart, whereas he considered the other boy "dumb," the idea of his transformation into the other boy caused him considerable anxiety. More recent obsessions were over things that he had said or done, whether they were "correct," and whether he would be "punished" if they were not. In addition, he could only cross streets at marked crosswalks, and he could not allow himself to look at a cross atop any church or other religious building. These behaviors reassured him that he would not be punished by God for any mistakes he may have made. Whenever he stopped eating, he had to announce to himself just before stopping that he had taken his last bite. More often than not, he would be uncertain that he had in fact done so, and thus he would continue to eat and stop, eat and stop. A similar ritual preoccupied him when attempting to get up from the toilet. Had he announced that he had wiped himself for the last time? These thoughts and rituals preoccupied him for much of the day and required immense amounts of mental effort to be pushed out of consciousness.

As mentioned earlier, activities such as eating, sex, gambling, or drinking can be done to excess and possibly meet criteria for a mental disorder. Such behaviors are not compulsions in the strict sense, because they give the person pleasure and are resisted only because of their secondary, deleterious consequences. The compulsions of OCD are never described as pleasurable and they evoke considerable effort on the part of the affected person to resist them, because they are inherently distressing and because they directly interfere with functioning.

Depressed patients frequently "obsess" about undesirable personal characteristics, negative life events or life circumstances, or "sins" of commission or omission about which they feel guilty. Such brooding or rumination is not, strictly speaking, obsessive, however, because it is rarely experienced as inappropriate or senseless, and it is mood-congruent. On the contrary, depressive rumination is most often meaningful, when considered in the person's immediate context.

Patients with obsessional fears of dirt or disease may develop phobic avoidance behaviors. Avoidance behaviors may become highly ritualized or stereotypic. In such cases, an additional diagnosis of a simple or specific phobia is not made according to DSM-III-R or DSM-IV criteria. Phobias usually require the presence of a feared object or situation to provoke anxiety and avoidance behavior (Stein and Hollander 1993) This is not so in OCD. The multiple unrealistic and excessive worries of generalized anxiety disorder may also resemble obsessions, but generalized anxiety disorder is ruled out if worries are limited to the concerns of comorbid OCD. Furthermore, the worries of generalized anxiety disorder are experienced as excessive concerns about real-life circumstances; obsessions are experienced as inappropriate because they do not typically involve realistic problems.

When an obsession is firmly held, it may become an overvalued idea, on a continuum with a delusion. In such cases, a psychotic disorder such as brief psychotic disorder, schizophreniform disorder, schizophrenia, or delusional disorder may need to be ruled out. Persons with typical OCD do not experience their obsessions as being imposed on them from the outside (as in thought insertion), do not have hallucinatory experiences, and can eventually recognize that their beliefs or fears are unfounded. Delusional disorders are more likely to have onset later in life than OCD, but in 10% to 20% of cases of apparent OCD, the obsessional ideas may become so fixed and ego-syntonic that they represent delusions (Insel and Akiskal 1986). The diagnoses of both OCD and delusional disorder or another psychotic disorder may be given if reality testing is lost and an obsession reaches delusional proportions. In DSM-IV, clinicians are instructed to specify "with poor insight" if a patient in a current episode of OCD does not recognize that the obsessions and compulsions are excessive or unreasonable.

Obsessive-compulsive disorder is equally common in men and women. Onset is usually in adolescence or early adulthood. OCD may co-occur with panic disorder, a depressive disorder (Rasmussen and Tsuang 1986), or a personality disorder (Skodol et al. 1995) (see discussion later in chapter). In these cases, more than one diagnosis will be warranted.

### Anorexia Nervosa

In contrast to bulimia nervosa, anorexia nervosa has features that are more consistently compulsive than impulsive. These include obsessive preoccupation with not gaining weight, compulsive dieting or exercise, and fixated disturbance in body image. In addition, patients with anorexia are typically rigid, meticulous, ritualistic, and perfectionistic (Kaye et al. 1993). If obsessions and compulsions are limited to ideas and behaviors related to eating and the body in a patient with anorexia nervosa, then the additional diagnosis of OCD is not made. If there are other obsessions or compulsions, both diagnoses may be warranted. Bulimia, however, can occur in association with anorexia nervosa, either concurrently or on lifetime history (Skodol et al. 1993). This suggests that patients with eating disorders may fall anywhere on the impulsive-compulsive spectrum and that some may shift along the spectrum over time. According to DSM-IV, if a person engages in binge eating or purging behavior during a period of anorexia nervosa, only the anorexia nervosa diagnosis is given, with a subtype designation of binge eating/purging type. Hudson and co-workers (1983) found a lifetime incidence of OCD of 69% in patients with "restrictor" anorexia nervosa and 44% in patients with "bulimic" anorexia nervosa.

Anorexia nervosa occurs predominantly in adolescent females. It may be associated with clinical depression (Hudson et al.

1983; Rothenberg 1988), although some of the physical signs and symptoms of anorexia may be misinterpreted as vegetative signs and symptoms of a depressive disorder (Strober and Katz 1988). Obsessive-compulsive personality traits are often thought to characterize the premorbid personalities of patients with anorexia nervosa (Holden 1990). In our own clinical research, we found a significantly elevated risk for avoidant personality disorder, but not obsessive-compulsive personality disorder, in patients with lifetime histories of anorexia nervosa (Skodol et al. 1993).

### Body Dysmorphic Disorder

Body dysmorphic disorder is characterized by preoccupation with an imagined or grossly exaggerated physical defect or anomaly in a normal-appearing person. The most common complaints of patients with body dysmorphic disorder are of facial flaws, such as wrinkles, spots, scars, vascular markings, acne, paleness or redness of the complexion, swelling, asymmetry or disproportion, and excessive hair. Other preoccupations may involve the shape, size, or other aspect of the facial or other anatomy, such as the nose, eyes, eyelids, eyebrows, ears, mouth, lips, teeth, jaw, chin, cheeks, head, genitals, breasts, buttocks, abdomen, arms, hands, feet, legs, hips, shoulders, spine, or skin (Phillips 1991). Body dysmorphic disorder occurs slightly more frequently in women than in men. Age at onset is usually from early adolescence through the 20s.

Several disorders should especially be considered in the differential diagnosis of body dysmorphic disorder (Table 1–4). Patients with anorexia nervosa imagine that they are fat, even when emaciated. The diagnosis of body dysmorphic disorder is not made if bodily concerns are better explained as anorexia nervosa. The symptoms of body dysmorphic disorder are similar to those of OCD. There are persistently or recurrently intrusive thoughts and images that are difficult to suppress or ignore. Patients frequently engage in compulsive, ritualistic behavior such as mirror checking. In fact, however, the ideas of the patient with body dysmorphic disorder usually are not as intrusive, or resisted as staunchly, as the obsessions in the patient with OCD, and they are not regarded as senseless. The diagnosis of OCD would not be made, in any case, if obsessions and compulsions are limited to the imagined defects of body dysmorphic disorder. If a person's bodily preoccupation concerns being of the wrong anatomical sex, a gender identity disorder is diagnosed, not body dysmorphic disorder. Patients with depressive disorders, social phobia, avoidant personalty disorder, or other disorders may also have concerns with defects in physical appearance. These concerns are not usually the predominant disturbance, however. Nevertheless, body dysmorphic disorder may be diagnosed in association with comorbid mood, anxiety, or personality disorders, if warranted.

Sometimes the ideas of body dysmorphic disorder are held with intense conviction. As such, they may become frank delusions. Historically, body dysmorphic disorder was classified as one of the monosymptomatic hypochondriacal psychoses (Bishop 1980), and a diagnosis of delusional disorder, somatic type may apply in some cases (deLeon et al. 1989). DSM-IV allows both diagnoses to be made, rather than providing for a subtype with delusions. At the other end of the spectrum, many apparently psychiatrically healthy people are dissatisfied with some aspect of their physical appearance, and large numbers seek surgical correction of the defects. Minimal objective evidence of disfigurement and unusual surgical requests may suggest body dysmorphic disorder, which in turn is likely to result in poor surgical outcome (Hollander and Phillips 1993).

The symptoms of body dysmorphic disorder illustrate how dysmorphophobia may be distributed along a continuum of severity, insight, or certainty of conviction, ranging from a preoccupation to an obsession, an overvalued idea, or a delusion (Phillips 1991). The degree of conviction (and thus the appropriate diagnosis) might vary over the course of the patient's illness or even as regards one defect versus another. The differential diagnosis of body dysmorphic disorder (Table 1–4) also illustrates how cognitive disinhibition (obsessions) and compensatory behavioral disinhibition (compulsions) can appear to be one mechanism affecting different aspects of self or behavior in different individuals or at different times.

**Table 1–4.** Disorders in the differential diagnosis of body dysmorphic disorder

| Disorder | Principal distinguishing feature(s) |
| --- | --- |
| Anorexia nervosa | Preoccupation with imagined defect in appearance limited to dissatisfaction with body shape and size |
| Obsessive-compulsive disorder | Ideas more intrusive, resisted more, and often regarded as senseless. Concerns not limited to imagined physical defects. |
| Gender identity disorder | Preoccupation with defect in physical appearance limited to discomfort with one's primary and secondary sex characteristics. |
| Delusional disorder, somatic type | Beliefs are delusional, that is, false beliefs based on incorrect inference about external reality and firmly sustained in spite of incontrovertible and obvious proof or evidence to the contrary. |
| Major depression | Concerns with physical appearance occur only in context of major depressive episode. |

Depersonalization disorder is similar to body dysmorphic disorder in that the affected patient has an obsessive preoccupation with an aspect of the body, in this case with perceived sensory alterations, and engages in compulsive checking behaviors (Hollander and Phillips 1993). Depersonalization is an alteration in the perception or experience of the self in which a person's usual sense of his or her own reality is temporarily lost or changed. The feeling is one of being detached or outside of one's body. This feeling is ego-dystonic, and reality testing is preserved.

Whether depersonalization occurs more in women or in men is controversial. Age at onset of depersonalization is in adolescence or early adulthood. The symptom of depersonalization can occur in other disorders, particularly psychotic disorders or panic disorder. When it occurs as a symptom of a more symptomatically pervasive disorder, a separate diagnosis is not needed. Premorbid obsessional personality has been observed in more than 75% of patients with depersonalization (Torch 1978).

**Hypochondriasis**

In hypochondriasis, there is preoccupation with the fear of having or belief in having a serious disease, based on a person's misinterpretation of physical signs or sensations, in the absence of a diagnosable physical disorder to account for the symptoms. Females outnumber males in samples of hypochondriacal patients. The disorder appears to be one of mid-adult life.

> A 28-year-old attorney sought a psychiatric consultation at the suggestion of her father, who was concerned about her undiagnosed physical complaints. The woman had graduated from law school 3 years previously and had been working successfully at a firm specializing in securities law in a city far from her family home. However, for the past year, she had felt "sick" on and off. Her physical symptoms were of exhaustion, headaches, dizziness, nausea, abdominal pain, and diarrhea. In addition, she was having trouble falling asleep. She had seen her internist, a neurologist, an ophthalmologist, and a rheumatologist, each on several occasions. There were no findings on physical examination, and laboratory testing, both routine and exotic, had found no evidence of disease. Chronic fatigue syndrome was mentioned (the patient was negative for Epstein-Barr virus), but the patient was convinced that she had lupus or another serious disease that was, as yet, undetected. Her preoccupation with her "illness" not only had her repeatedly consulting with doctors and receiving more and more extensive and invasive workups, but was making it impossible for her to concentrate on her work, so that she was contemplating taking a leave of absence.

Typically, the fears of hypochondriasis are not as intrusive as the obsessions of OCD and are surely not regarded as senseless. Hypochondriasis, like body dysmorphic disorder and OCD, may also involve a spectrum of impairment of insight that ranges from obsessional ego-dystonic beliefs to delusional ego-syntonic convictions (Insel and Akiskal 1986) The compulsive behavior of seeking the reassurance of doctors through repeated consultations and evaluations is not stereotypic, as are the compulsive rituals of OCD. Nonetheless, similarities between hypochondriasis and OCD exist. Furthermore, hypochondriacal patients may have other obsessions and compulsions not involving illness, and patients with OCD diagnosed on other bases may have concerns about disease. With respect to the differential diagnosis between hypochondriasis and OCD, if the content of obsessions is limited to the fear of having disease in a patient with hypochondriasis, a diagnosis of OCD would not be made. If obsessions or compulsions are unrelated to hypochondriacal concerns, both diagnoses could apply. On the other hand, persistent thoughts about getting ill, rather than of actually being ill, are more consistent with OCD than hypochondriasis (Fallon et al. 1991). Fear of illness in general might represent a specific phobia. Patients with panic disorder are often convinced that they are having heart attacks (Noyes et al. 1986). Hypochondriacal concerns should not be limited to the symptoms of panic attacks and their interpretation. Typical hypochondriacal patients are more often concerned with having less-acute, life-threatening disorders, such as leukemia and AIDS (Fallon et al. 1993). Hypochondriasis may be a facet of somatization disorder. In hypochondriasis, the fear or belief in having a disease is the primary concern; in somatization disorder, the patient's focus is on the multiple, unexplained physical symptoms (Skodol 1989).

Hypochondriacal concerns can be found in patients with a variety of other mental disorders, including major depression or dysthymia, panic disorder, simple phobia, OCD, generalized anxiety disorder, somatization disorder, psychotic disorders, and personality disorders (Fallon et al. 1993). In fact, hypochondriasis has rarely been found in the absence of other diagnosable psychopathology. In a study by Barsky and co-workers (1992), 79% of 42 hypochondriacal patients were diagnosed with one or more concurrent Axis I disorders: 33% with major depression, 45% with dysthymia, 33% with phobias, 21% with generalized anxiety disorder, and 21% with somatization. Comorbidity was even greater on a lifetime basis; only 12% had no other lifetime Axis I diagnosis.

**Trichotillomania**

Trichotillomania is characterized by recurrent pulling out of one's own hair, resulting in noticeable hair loss. Common areas of the body for hair pulling are the scalp, eyebrows, eyelashes, and beard. The hair pulling and disposal of hair may be accompanied by specific rituals including mouthing or eating the hair.

Trichotillomania was added as a specific diagnosis to DSM-III-R and classified as an impulse-control disorder not elsewhere classified. The person with trichotillomania experiences an increasing sense of tension before hair pulling or in association with attempts to resist the urge, and gratification or a sense of relief during or after hair pulling. Although typically pleasurable, hair pulling is sometimes described as ego-dystonic and is resisted. The irresistible urge to pluck out hairs has been described as "compulsive" (Swedo 1993). The classification of trichotillomania as an impulse-control disorder has become controversial as similarities between it and OCD have been found. Patients seeking treatment for trichotillomania, like those seeking treatment for OCD, frequently do so because of distress and disability resulting from indulging in the behavior for several hours each day.

In contrast to OCD, however, hair pulling in trichotillomania is not purposeful or intentional and is not performed in response to an obsessional thought. Nor is hair pulling designed to prevent or neutralize discomfort (other than the anxiety associated with resisting) or some dreaded event or situation. Patients with trichotillomania persist in one behavior rather than changing rituals over time, as patients with OCD often do. The sex ratio for trichotillomania is different from the sex ratio for OCD: more females than males report compulsive hair pulling. Similarities and differences between trichotillomania and OCD are summarized in Table 1–5.

Axis I disorders that can be comorbid with trichotillomania include depressive disorders, generalized anxiety disorder, and substance use disorders. Axis II disorders that can be comorbid with trichotillomania include histrionic, borderline, and passive-aggressive personality disorders (Swedo 1993).

**Table 1–5.**   Comparison of trichotillomania and obsessive-compulsive disorder (OCD)

| Characteristic | Trichotillomania | OCD |
|---|---|---|
| Age at onset | Usually childhood | Usually adolescence or early adulthood |
| Sex ratio | More common in females | Equally common in males and females |
| Stereotyped behaviors | Yes | Yes |
| Driven quality | Yes | Yes |
| Pleasure, gratification, or relief from behavior | Yes | No |
| Purposeful behaviors | No | Yes |
| In response to obsessional thoughts | No | Yes |
| Designed to prevent dreaded event or situation | No | Yes |
| Associated disability | Yes | Yes |

## Axis II Disorders

### Borderline Personality Disorder

The diagnostic criteria for borderline personality disorder include items describing suicidal or self-mutilating behavior, other potentially self-damaging impulsiveness (e.g., overspending, indiscriminate sex, substance use, shoplifting, reckless driving, binge eating), and certain interpersonal behaviors that might indicate difficulties with impulsivity (e.g., rapid shifts in feelings toward others, frantic efforts to avoid abandonment). Borderline personality disorder would be expected to show high associations with Axis I disorders of impulse control because of overlapping criteria. Are these associations artifactual or real?

In making the diagnosis of borderline personality disorder in association with another impulse-control disorder, it is important that the general criteria for a personality disorder are met. The pattern of behavior should be pervasive, persistent over time, and exhibited with many people in many different contexts. The distress or impairment associated should not be limited to periods when an Axis I disorder is present.

Borderline personality disorder has been shown by several investigators to be associated with substance use disorders (Links et al. 1988; Zanarini et al. 1989) and bulimia (Herzog et al. 1992; Skodol et al. 1993), even with the overlapping items removed from the criteria set. These findings have led Zanarini (1993) to reconceptualize BPD as an impulsive spectrum disorder rather than an affective spectrum disorder. Borderline personality disorder may also co-occur with psychotic, mood, anxiety, or other personality disorders.

**Antisocial Personality Disorder**

Patients with antisocial personality disorder have a history of childhood conduct problems, many of which involve poor impulse control (e.g., starting fights, vandalizing property, setting fires). In addition, there are adult criteria for impulsivity or failure to plan ahead, irritability and aggressiveness, reckless disregard for safety, and consistent irresponsibility.

Although antisocial personality disorder and borderline personality disorder may be thought to differ on the interpersonal dimension—the person with antisocial personality disorder is "anti"-social, whereas the person with borderline personality disorder is intensely "social"—they may and do occur together. The two other disorders from Cluster B (the dramatic, emotional, or erratic cluster), histrionic and narcissistic personality disorders, may also co-occur (Oldham et al. 1992).

**Obsessive-Compulsive Personality Disorder**

On the compulsive end of the impulsive-compulsive spectrum on Axis II is obsessive-compulsive personality disorder. Compulsive overcontrol is evident in the diagnostic criteria of obsessive-compulsive personality disorder pertaining to perfectionism; preoccupation with lists, details, and order; and overconscientiousness. Overcontrol can also be interpreted from the rigidity and stubbornness of the person with obsessive-compulsive personality disorder and his or her need to have others do things exactly the way he or she does them or would want them done.

Traditionally, and in current nosology, obsessive-compulsive personality disorder is distinguished from OCD by the absence of ego-dystonic obsessions and compulsions. As stated above, however, distinctions based on the ego-syntonic/ego-dystonic nature of obsessive-compulsive symptoms are not always clear-cut. Although initially OCD and obsessive-compulsive personality disorder were thought to be related, results of comorbidity studies have been inconsistent (Skodol et al. 1995).

Obsessive-compulsive personality disorder and borderline personality disorder would seem to be at opposite ends of a spectrum. However, more recent data (Skodol and Oldham 1992) suggest that these disorders may co-occur. This finding seems consistent only if patients are viewed as shifting back and forth on the dimension of control, sometimes acting out and sometimes compensating with overcontrol. In this way, obsessive-compulsive personality disorder may be a general adaptational style designed to manage the impulsivity evident in borderline personality disorder. The specific and more limited compulsive behaviors of OCD, which are in response to disinhibited obsessional thoughts and are meant to control or compensate for them, would have an analogous function, although they do not represent a general adaptational style.

# Conclusions

It is evident that traditional distinctions between disorders that may constitute an impulsive-compulsive spectrum are often either arbitrary or difficult to make, or both. Indeed, the distinction between impulsivity and compulsivity itself seems blurred. If a spectrum of impulsive and compulsive disorders exists, it seems unlikely to be a simple, unidimensional one, but, instead, might involve interactions between several biological or psychological systems, each contributing to the varied presentations of psychopathology. The resulting disorder may be a function of a person's gender; aspect of mental processes, behavior, or functioning affected; severity of disturbance; stage of illness; or attempt at adaptation.

Virtually all of the disorders in the impulsive-compulsive spectrum have their onset in childhood, adolescence, or early adult life. For a number of the disorders, gender differences appear to exist. Eating disorders and other disorders involving physical appearance and health tend to be more common among females. Disorders involving sexual activities, aggression, and artificial alteration in states of consciousness (i.e., by drugs) are more common in males. These gender differences may reflect biological differences between the sexes or differences in socialization and role modeling. Comorbidity with other mental disorders is unusually high. In some cases, comorbid disorders appear to act as risk factors for the development of an impulsive-compulsive spectrum disorder; in other cases, comorbid disorders seem to be complications of disturbances of behavioral control, which often run a chronic course through early adulthood. The course of impulsive and compulsive disorders in later life is unknown, although there are some suggestions that impulsive behaviors may become attenuated with advancing age.

Productive next steps would include study of patterns of comorbidity among disorders thought to occupy the spectrum so as to search for related disorders that might share fundamental dimensions of disturbance. Lifetime versus concurrent comorbidity should be distinguished, and the relationship of impulsive-compulsive spectrum disorders to one another and to other mental disorders over time should be determined. Measuring personality traits and other psychopathology dimensionally will help to quantify differences between apparently related conditions. Multifaceted biological studies should be directed at groups of disorders sharing common psychopathological disturbances. Likewise, treatment studies should be targeted at empirically derived dimensions of psychopathology.

# References

Abel GG, Becker JV, Cunningham-Rathner J, et al: Multiple paraphilic diagnoses among sex offenders. Bull Am Acad Psychiatry Law 16:153–168, 1988

American Psychiatric Association: Diagnostic and Statistical Manual of Mental Disorders, 3rd Edition. Washington, DC, American Psychiatric Association, 1980

American Psychiatric Association: Diagnostic and Statistical Manual of Mental Disorders, 3rd Edition, Revised. Washington, DC, American Psychiatric Association, 1987

American Psychiatric Association: Diagnostic and Statistical Manual of Mental Disorders, 4th Edition. Washington, DC, American Psychiatric Association, 1994

Anthony DT, Hollander E: Sexual compulsions, in Obsessive-Compulsive–Related Disorders. Edited by Hollander E. Washington, DC, American Psychiatric Press, 1993, pp 139–150

Barsky AJ, Wyshak G, Klerman GL: Psychiatric comorbidity in DSM-III-R hypochondriasis. Arch Gen Psychiatry 49:101–108, 1992

Bishop ER: Monosymptomatic hypochondriasis. Psychosomatics 21: 731–747, 1980

Christenson GA, MacKenzie TB, Mitchell JE: Characteristics of 60 adult chronic hair pullers. Am J Psychiatry 148:365–370, 1991

Coleman E: Is your patient suffering from compulsive sexual behavior? Psychiatric Annals 22:320–325, 1992

Cummings JL: Clinical Neuropsychiatry. Orlando, FL, Grune & Stratton, 1985

deLeon J, Bott A, Simpson GM: Dysmorphophobia: body dysmorphic disorder or delusional disorder, somatic subtype? Compr Psychiatry 30:457–472, 1989

Fallon BA, Javitch JA, Hollander E, et al: Hypochondriasis and obsessive compulsive disorder: overlaps in diagnosis and treatment. J Clin Psychiatry 52:457–460, 1991

Fallon BA, Rasmussen SA, Liebowitz MR: Hypochondriasis, in Obsessive-Compulsive–Related Disorders. Edited by Hollander E. Washington, DC, American Psychiatric Press, 1993, pp 71–92

Fogel BS, Stone AB: Practical pathophysiology in neuropsychiatry: a clinical approach to depression and impulsive behavior in neurological patients, in The American Psychiatric Press Textbook of Neuropsychiatry, 2nd Edition. Edited by Yudofsky SC, Hales RE. Washington, DC, American Psychiatric Press, 1992, pp 329–344

Herzog DB, Keller MB, Lavori PW, et al: The prevalence of personality disorders in 210 women with eating disorders. J Clin Psychiatry 53:147–152, 1992

Holden NL: Is anorexia nervosa an obsessive-compulsive disorder? Br J Psychiatry 157:1–5, 1990

Hollander E: Introduction, in Obsessive-Compulsive–Related Disorders. Edited by Hollander E. Washington, DC, American Psychiatric Press, 1993, pp 1–16

Hollander E, Phillips KA: Body image and experience disorders, in Obsessive-Compulsive–Related Disorders. Edited by Hollander E. Washington, DC, American Psychiatric Press, 1993, pp 17–48

Hudson JI Jr, Pope HG Jr, Jonas JM, et al: Phenomenologic relationships of eating disorders to major affective disorder. Psychiatry Res 9:345–354, 1983

Insel TR, Akiskal HS: Obsessive-compulsive disorder with psychotic features: a phenomenological analysis. Am J Psychiatry 143:1527–1533, 1986

Katz JL: Eating disorders and substance abuse disorders, in American Psychiatric Press Review of Psychiatry, Vol 11. Edited by Tasman A, Riba MB. Washington, DC, American Psychiatric Press, 1992, pp 436–452

Kaye WH, Weltzin T, Hsu LKG: Anorexia nervosa, in Obsessive-Compulsive–Related Disorders. Edited by Hollander E. Washington, DC, American Psychiatric Press, 1993, pp 49–70

Leckman JF: Tourette's syndrome, in Obsessive-Compulsive–Related Disorders. Edited by Hollander E. Washington, DC, American Psychiatric Press, 1993, pp 113–137

Linden RD, Pope HG Jr, Jonas JM: Pathological gambling and major affective disorder: preliminary findings. J Clin Psychiatry 47:201–203, 1986

Links PS, Steiner M, Offord DR, et al: Characteristics of borderline personality disorder: a Canadian study. Can J Psychiatry 33:336–340, 1988

Mannuzza S, Klein RG, Bessler A, et al: Adult outcome of hyperactive boys: educational achievement, occupational rank, and psychiatric status. Arch Gen Psychiatry 50:565–576, 1993

McElroy SL, Pope HG Jr, Hudson JI Jr, et al: Kleptomania: a report of 20 cases. Am J Psychiatry 148:652–657, 1991

McElroy SL, Hudson JI Jr, Pope HG Jr, et al: The DSM-III-R impulse control disorders not elsewhere classified: clinical characteristics and relationship to other psychiatric disorders. Am J Psychiatry 149:318–327, 1992

Money J: Lovemaps: Clinical Concepts of Sexually Erotic Health and Pathology, Paraphilia, and Gender Transposition in Childhood, Adolescence, and Maturity. New York, Irvington Publishers, 1986

Noyes R, Reich J, Clancy J: Reduction in hypochondriasis with treatment of panic disorder. Am J Psychiatry 149:631–635, 1986

Oldham JM, Skodol AE, Kellman HD, et al: Diagnosis of DSM-III-R personality disorders: patterns of comorbidity by two structured interviews. Am J Psychiatry 149:213–220, 1992

Ovsiew F: Bedside neuropsychiatry: eliciting the clinical phenomena of neuropsychiatric illness, in The American Psychiatric Press Textbook of Neuropsychiatry, 2nd Edition. Edited by Yudofsky SC, Hales RE. Washington, DC, American Psychiatric Press, 1992, pp 89–125

Phillips KA: Body dysmorphic disorder: the distress of imagined ugliness. Am J Psychiatry 148:1138–1149, 1991

Qualand MC: Compulsive sexual behavior: definition of a problem and an approach to treatment. J Sex Marital Ther 11:121–132, 1985

Ramirez LF, McCormick RA, Russo AM, et al: Patterns of substance abuse in pathological gamblers undergoing treatment. Addict Behav 8:425–428, 1983

Rasmussen SA, Tsuang MT: Clinical characteristics and family history in DSM-III obsessive-compulsive disorder. Am J Psychiatry 143:317–322, 1986

Rothenberg A: Differential diagnosis of anorexia nervosa and depressive illness: a review of 11 studies. Compr Psychiatry 29:427–432, 1988

Roy A, Adinoff B, Roehrich L, et al: Pathological gambling: a psychobiological study. Arch Gen Psychiatry 45:369–373, 1988

Skodol AE: Problems in Differential Diagnosis: From DSM-III to DSM-III-R in Clinical Practice. Washington, DC, American Psychiatric Press, 1989

Skodol AE, Oldham JM: Impulsivity/compulsivity: differential diagnosis. Paper presented at the 145th annual meeting of the American Psychiatric Association, Washington, DC, May 1992

Skodol AE, Oldham JM, Hyler SE, et al: Comorbidity of DSM-III-R eating disorders and personality disorders. Int J Eat Disord 14:403–416, 1993

Skodol AE, Oldham JM, Hyler SE, et al: Patterns of anxiety and personality disorder comorbidity. J Psychiatr Res 29:361–374, 1995

Sprenkle DH: Treating a sex addict through marital sex therapy. Family Relations 36:11–14, 1987

Stein DJ, Hollander E: The spectrum of obsessive-compulsive–related disorders, in Obsessive-Compulsive–Related Disorders. Edited by Hollander E. Washington, DC, American Psychiatric Press, 1993, pp 241–271

Strober M, Katz JL: Depression in the eating disorders: a review and analysis of descriptive, family, and biological findings, in Diagnostic Issues in Anorexia Nervosa and Bulimia Nervosa. Edited by Garner DM, Garfinkel PE. New York, Brunner/Mazel, 1988, pp 80–111

Swedo SE: Trichotillomania, in Obsessive-Compulsive–Related Disorders. Edited by Hollander E. Washington, DC, American Psychiatric Press, 1993, pp 93–111

Swedo SE, Leonard HL, Rapoport JL, et al: A double-blind comparison of clomipramine and desipramine in the treatment of trichotillomania (hair-pulling). N Engl J Med 321:497–501, 1989

Torch E: Review of the relationship between obsession and depersonalization. Acta Psychiatr Scand 58:191–198, 1978

Weissberg JH, Levay AN: Compulsive sexual behavior. Medical Aspects of Human Sexuality 20:129–132, 1986

Wender PH, Reimherr FW, Wood DR: Attention deficit disorder ("minimal brain dysfunction") in adults: a replication study of diagnosis and drug treatment. Arch Gen Psychiatry 38:449–456, 1981

Woods DJ: Carving nature at its joints? Observations on a revised psychiatric nomenclature. J Clin Psychol 35:912–920, 1979

World Health Organization: International Classification of Diseases, 10th Revision. Geneva, World Health Organization, 1992

Zanarini MC: Borderline personality disorder as an impulse spectrum disorder, in Borderline Personality Disorder: Etiology and Treatment. Edited by Paris J. Washington, DC, American Psychiatric Press, 1993, pp 67–85

Zanarini MC, Gunderson JG, Frankenburg FR: Axis I phenomenology of borderline personality disorder. Compr Psychiatry 30:149–156, 1989

# 2

# Borderline Personality Disorder: Impulsive and Compulsive Features

## Mary C. Zanarini, Ed.D.
## Elizabeth Weinberg, M.D.

---

J enike (1990) was the first modern author to suggest that there is a spectrum of disorders related to obsessive-compulsive disorder (OCD). He listed the following as *OCD spectrum disorders* or perhaps attenuated or subthreshold forms of OCD: trichotillomania, pathological gambling, monosymptomatic hypochondriasis and dysmorphophobia, globus hystericus, obsessive fear of AIDS, bowel obsessions, urinary obsessions, compulsive face picking, compulsive water drinking, anorexia nervosa, and compulsive self-mutilation.

More recently, there has been much interest in the psychopathological dimensions of compulsivity and impulsivity. Hollander and colleagues (Hollander 1993; Stein and Hollander 1993) have suggested that compulsivity and impulsivity represent two ends of a continuum of restraint versus disinhibition. These authors suggest that OCD is the prototypic compulsive disorder and that borderline personality disorder (BPD) is the prototypic impulsive disorder. They also suggest that there is a family of obsessive-compulsive–related or spectrum disorders and include among these disorders the following: OCD, body dysmorphic disorder, depersonalization disorder, anorexia nervosa, hypochondriasis, trichotillomania, Tourette's disorder, sexual compulsions, pathological gambling, and impulsive personality disorders (BPD and antisocial personality disorder).

McElroy and colleagues (1992, 1993) have suggested that compulsivity and impulsivity may represent different dimensions of psychopathology and that these dimensions may intersect or be orthogonal to one another. In either case, these authors have hypothesized that a number of disorders are impulse spectrum disorders and include among these disorders the following: intermittent explosive disorder, kleptomania, pathological gambling, pyromania, trichotillomania, anorexia nervosa, bulimia nervosa, alcohol abuse and dependence, drug abuse and dependence, antisocial personality disorder, and BPD.

The place of BPD in psychiatric nosology has long been a point of contention. Stern (1938) was the first author to use the term "borderline" to describe a specific pathological condition—a condition that he thought had both neurotic and psychotic features. Since that time, there have been six main conceptualizations of this term.

The first of these conceptualizations is based on the work of Kernberg (1975). In this view, the term borderline is used to describe most serious forms of character pathology. The second conceptualization reflects the work of Gunderson (1984). In this view, the term borderline describes a specific form of personality disorder that can be distinguished from a substantial number of other Axis II disorders, particularly those in the "odd" and "anxious" clusters of DSM-III (American Psychiatric Association 1980) and DSM-III-R (American Psychiatric Association 1987). The third conceptualization, which flourished in the 1960s and 1970s, focused on the propensity of borderline patients to have transient psychotic or psychotic-like experiences. In this view, borderline personality was thought of as being a schizophrenia spectrum disorder (Wender 1977). The fourth of these conceptualizations, which was the organizing construct for much of the clinical care and empirical research in the 1980s, focused on the chronic dysphoria and affective lability of borderline patients. In this view, borderline personality was thought of as an affective spectrum disorder (Akiskal 1981; Stone 1980).

Both the fifth and sixth conceptualizations of borderline psychopathology have arisen during the 1990s. Zanarini and colleagues (1993) have proposed that BPD is best conceptualized as an impulse spectrum disorder (i.e., a disorder related to substance use disorders, antisocial personality disorder, and perhaps eating disorders). In this view, BPD is not seen as an attenuated or atypical form of one of these impulse spectrum disorders. Rather, these authors suggest that BPD is a specific form of personality disorder that may share a propensity to action with other disorders of impulse control.

During the late 1980s and early 1990s, six studies reported that a history of physical and sexual abuse was relatively common among patients with criteria-defined BPD and that sexual abuse was significantly more common among borderline patients than among depressed control subjects or control subjects with personality disorders (Herman et al. 1989; Links et al. 1988; Ogata et al. 1990; Shearer et al. 1990; Westen et al. 1990; Zanarini et al. 1989c). These reports served as the empirical basis for the sixth conceptualization of BPD—that of BPD as a trauma spectrum disorder, related to PTSD and dissociative disorders, including multiple personality disorder (dissociative identity disorder).

Until very recently, there was little theoretical interest in or empirical support for a relationship between BPD and obsessive-compulsive spectrum disorders. However, Skodol and colleagues (Oldham et al. 1992; Skodol et al. 1994) have recently found a substantial prevalence of OCD and obsessive-compulsive personality disorder in two related samples of patients with criteria-defined BPD.

In this chapter we review the literature concerning the phenomenology of BPD to assess the relationship between BPD and compulsive and impulsive spectrum disorders. Data from a recent study of the phenomenology of patients with criteria-defined BPD are presented. We detail data from the realms of both syndromal (i.e., Axis I and Axis II disorders) and subsyndromal (i.e., symptoms, symptom clusters, and personality traits) phenomenology. We then describe alternative ways of understanding the relationship between borderline psychopathology and both of these spectra of disorders and dimensions of psychopathology.

## Axis I and Axis II Phenomenology of Borderline Personality Disorder

To date, nine studies that have assessed a range of Axis I and Axis II disorders in the histories of patients with criteria-defined BPD have been published. Taken together, the findings suggest that BPD bears little relation to schizophrenia spectrum disorders in the realm of phenomenology. These studies also suggest that the relationship between BPD and affective spectrum disorders is strong but not specific, as most control groups studied also exhibited high rates of affective disorder (see Zanarini 1993 for a review of the relationship between BPD and disorders on these spectra).

The relationship between BPD and both compulsive and impulsive spectrum disorders, as characterized by comorbidity studies, is detailed in Table 2–1. For the purposes of this review, compulsive spectrum disorders include OCD, (obsessive) compulsive personality disorder, hypochondriasis, and "pure" anorexia nervosa, and impulse spectrum disorders include substance use disorders, other eating disorders ("pure" bulimia nervosa and mixed anorexia/bulimia), and antisocial personality disorder.

In the first of these nine studies, Akiskal (1981) studied 100 consecutive outpatients at two urban mental health centers in Tennessee who met at least five of the six Gunderson-Singer criteria for BPD (Gunderson and Singer 1975). Each of these patients also met the DSM-III criteria for BPD. A semistructured interview was administered by a research psychiatrist to obtain phenom-

**Table 2–1.** Compulsive and impulsive spectrum disorders: comorbidity studies

| Study | BPD (n) | OCD | Hypo-chondriasis | Anorexia | Other eating disturbance[a] | CPD | Substance abuse[b] | APD |
|---|---|---|---|---|---|---|---|---|
| Akiskal (1981) | 100 | 8.0 | 0.0 | 0.0 | 0.0 | 0.0 | 57.0 | 13.0 |
| McGlashan and Heinssen (1989)[c] | 58 | — | — | — | — | — | — | 31.0 |
| Pope et al. (1983) | 33 | 0.0 | 0.0 | 3.0 | 0.0 | 0.0 | 67.0 | 9.0 |
| Andrulonis and Vogel (1984) | 106 | — | — | 29.0[d] | 29.0[d] | — | 69.0 | 69.0[e] |
| Frances et al. (1984) | 26 | — | — | 0.0 | 0.0 | 0.0 | 23.0 | 0.0 |
| Perry and Cooper (1985) | 23 | — | — | — | — | — | 43.0 / 87.0 | 25.5[f] |
| Links et al. (1988) | 88 | 8.3 | — | — | — | 0.0 | 31.4 / 22.9 | 13.1 |
| Zanarini et al. (1989a) | 50 | 0.0 | 0.0 | 6.0 | 8.0 | 2.0 | 66.0 / 70.0 | 60.0 |
| Coid (1993) | 72[g] | 15.0 | 0.0 | 6.0 | 0.0 | 10.0 | 42.0 / 36.0 | 49.0 |

*Note.* BPD = borderline personality disorder; OCD = obsessive-compulsive disorder; CPD = compulsive personality disorder; APD = antisocial personality disorder.

[a] Bulimia nervosa or anorexia/bulimia nervosa.
[b] In those rows with two entries, the top figure pertains to alcohol abuse and the bottom figure pertains to drug abuse.
[c] Significant antisocial traits.
[d] Both obesity and anorexia are included in the 29%.
[e] Substantial antisocial acting out.
[f] Pertains to definite and trait borderline patients combined.
[g] All female sample.

enological information according to DSM-III criteria. Using this information, Akiskal then made all Axis I and Axis II diagnoses that were applicable. He found that 57% of his borderline cohort met the criteria for a substance use disorder, 13% met the criteria for antisocial personality disorder, and 8% met the criteria for OCD. No patients were reported to have met the criteria for hypochondriasis, an eating disorder, or compulsive personality disorder.

McGlashan (1983) studied the Axis I phenomenology of a retrospectively diagnosed sample of inpatients who met the Diagnostic Interview for Borderlines (DIB; Gunderson et al. 1981) ($n = 82$) and/or DSM-III criteria for BPD ($n = 97$). A research team reviewed the charts of all patients discharged from Chestnut Lodge between 1950 and 1975 who 1) were between 16 and 55 years of age on admission, 2) had a hospitalization of at least 90 days, and 3) were not suffering from an organic brain syndrome. In a study of a subsample of the same cohort, McGlashan and Heinssen (1989) found that none of 58 patients with DIB- and/or DSM-III–defined BPD met the DSM-III criteria for antisocial personality disorder, but that 31% had significant antisocial traits.

Pope and colleagues (1983) studied the Axis I and Axis II phenomenology of a group of 33 inpatients at McLean Hospital who met the DSM-III criteria for BPD. An investigator reviewed the charts of 39 patients who had previously been given a clinical or DIB diagnosis of BPD and determined which of them met the DSM-III criteria for this disorder. Pope and colleagues found that 67% of the sample met the criteria for some type of substance use disorder, 9% met the criteria for antisocial personality disorder, and 3% met the criteria for anorexia nervosa. They also found that none of their cohort met the DSM-III criteria for OCD, hypochondriasis, compulsive personality disorder, or bulimia nervosa.

Andrulonis and Vogel (1984) studied the phenomenology of three groups of inpatients at the Institute of Living who met the DSM-III criteria for the following disorders: nonschizotypal BPD ($n = 106$), schizophrenia ($n = 55$), and some form of affective disorder (bipolar disorder [$n = 4$], major depression [$n = 32$], and dysthymic disorder [$n = 19$]). These diagnoses were made by a research psychiatrist on the basis of a clinical interview and chart review. None of the patients with BPD was currently suffering from a major affective disorder, and none of the control patients (i.e., those with schizophrenia or affective disorder) had a concurrent Axis II diagnosis. In addition, no patient had an IQ of less than 80 or a primary diagnosis other than BPD, schizophrenia, or an affective disorder. Phenomenological data, which were collected through a chart review, had to be well documented by past psychiatric or legal records. Andrulonis and Vogel found that 69% of their borderline cohort had engaged in antisocial acting out (i.e., violence toward property or others, criminal acts, promiscuity, and/or running away), 69% had a history of serious substance abuse, and 29% had a history of an eating disturbance (significant obesity of several years' duration or anorexia resulting in significant weight loss). These authors also found that borderline patients were significantly more likely than those in either control group to have engaged in both antisocial acting out and to have a history of substance abuse.

Frances and associates (1984) studied 76 outpatients between the ages of 18 and 45 at the Payne Whitney Evaluation Service who were thought to meet the criteria for an Axis II disorder but not to be suffering from a psychotic or organic disorder. After a 1-hour clinical interview performed conjointly by one to three raters, all appropriate Axis I and Axis II diagnoses were made. Twenty-six patients met the DSM-III criteria for BPD, while 46 of the remaining 50 patients (the control group) met the DSM-III criteria for at least one nonborderline form of personality disorder. Frances and associates found that 23% of the patients with BPD met the criteria for a substance use disorder and 8% met the criteria for an anxiety and/or somatoform disorder (specific type unspecified). These authors also found that none of the borderline patients met the DSM-III criteria for an eating disorder or compulsive and/or antisocial personality disorder. In addition, no between-group comparisons significantly discriminated the borderline patients from the control subjects.

Perry and Cooper (1985) studied the syndromal phenomenology of a group of 82 outpatients, symptomatic volunteers, and probationers from the metropolitan Boston area. After participating in a lengthy semistructured diagnostic interview, the sample was divided into the following five groups: definite BPD ($n = 23$), BPD trait ($n = 14$), antisocial personality disorder ($n = 14$), BPD and APD ($n = 12$), and bipolar II disorder ($n = 19$). After the initial interview was conducted, trained research assistants administered the Diagnostic Interview Schedule (Robins et al. 1981), a structured interview designed to assess the lifetime prevalence of various psychiatric disorders. Perry and Cooper found that 43% of their definite BPD group had a history of alcohol abuse and/or dependence and that 87% met the DSM-III criteria for drug abuse and/or dependence. However, both alcohol abuse/dependence and drug abuse/dependence were also common among antisocial and bipolar II patients, and no significant between-group differences were found. In addition, 25.5% of the patients with definite BPD or trait BPD met the DSM-III criteria for antisocial personality disorder.

Links and colleagues (1988) screened consecutive inpatients who met three or more of the seven best indicators for BPD (Gunderson and Kolb 1978). Patients were excluded if they met any of the following exclusion criteria: 1) a primary diagnosis of alcoholism or drug dependence, 2) organicity based on clinical evidence of a CNS abnormality of any etiology, 3) any physical disorders of known psychiatric significance, 4) borderline mental retardation, 5) a history of hospitalization for more than 2 years cumulatively of the previous 5, and 6) inability to understand English. The remaining 130 patients were interviewed with the DIB and the Schedule for Affective Disorders and Schizophrenia (Endicott and Spitzer 1978), which assesses disorders according to Research Diagnostic Criteria (RDC; Spitzer et al. 1978). Eighty-eight of these patients met the DIB criteria for BPD, whereas 42 borderline trait control subjects did not. In terms of lifetime diagnoses, 31.4% of the borderline patients met the RDC criteria for alcoholism, 22.9% met the RDC criteria for drug abuse, 13.1% met the RDC criteria for antisocial personality disorder, and 8.3% met the RDC criteria for OCD. Prevalence rates of eating disorders, obsessive-compulsive personality disorder, and hypochondriasis were not assessed.

No significant differences emerged between the borderline patients and the borderline trait control subjects.

Zanarini and associates (1988, 1989a) studied the lifetime Axis I and Axis II phenomenology of 50 borderline patients meeting both the Revised Diagnostic Interview for Borderlines (DIB-R; Zanarini et al. 1989b) and DSM-III criteria for BPD using the Structured Clinical Interview for DSM-III Axis I Disorders (Spitzer and Williams 1984) and the Diagnostic Interview for Personality Disorders (Zanarini et al. 1987a). They also studied the lifetime syndromal phenomenology of 29 control subjects with antisocial personality disorder and 26 control subjects who met the DSM-III criteria for dysthymic disorder and the DSM-III criteria for a nonborderline and nonantisocial form of personality disorder. All patients met the following inclusion criteria: 1) age between 18 and 40, 2) average or better intelligence, and 3) no history or current symptomatology of a clear-cut organic condition or major psychotic disorder (i.e., schizophrenia or bipolar disorder). Zanarini and associates found that 70% of the patients with BPD had met DSM-III criteria for drug abuse/dependence, 66% had met the DSM-III criteria for alcohol abuse/dependence, 60% had met the DSM-III criteria for antisocial personality disorder, and 8% had met the DSM-III criteria for bulimia nervosa. They also found that no borderline patients had met the DSM-III criteria for OCD or hypochondriasis, only 2% had met the DSM-III criteria for compulsive personality disorder, and just 6% had met the DSM-III criteria for anorexia nervosa. When compared with control subjects, borderline patients were significantly more likely than control subjects with dysthymic disorder and a nonborderline and nonantisocial form of personality disorder and significantly less likely than antisocial control subjects to have met the DSM-III criteria for alcohol abuse/dependence, drug abuse/dependence, and antisocial personality disorder.

Coid (1993) studied the Axis I and Axis II phenomenology of 72 female inpatients in England who met the DSM-III criteria for BPD using the Diagnostic Interview Schedule and the Structured Clinical Interview for DSM-III Axis II Disorders (Spitzer and Williams 1983). He found that 42% of his sample met lifetime criteria for alcohol abuse/dependence, 36% met the criteria for drug abuse/dependence, 15% met the criteria for OCD, and 6% met the criteria for anorexia nervosa. He also found that 10% of his sample met the criteria for compulsive personality disorder and 49% met the criteria for antisocial personality disorder.

# Recent Empirical Data Relating to the Compulsive and Impulsive Aspects of Borderline Psychopathology

The study described in this section began as one site in the DSM-IV Axis II Field Trials but evolved into a larger study of the validity of BPD as a diagnostic entity.

## Study Sample and Methodology

In this study, 136 inpatients at McLean Hospital in Belmont, Massachusetts, were interviewed concerning all aspects of their phenomenology as well as their family history of psychiatric disorder and childhood experiences. More specifically, each patient was initially screened to determine that he or she 1) was between the ages of 18 and 60, 2) had average or better intelligence, 3) had no history or current symptomatology of a serious organic condition or major psychotic disorder (i.e., schizophrenia or bipolar disorder), and 4) had been given a definite or probable Axis II diagnosis by the admitting physician. Written informed consent for participation in the study was obtained from each patient. Three semi-structured diagnostic interviews were then administered to each patient by one of four diagnosticians: a board-certified psychiatrist, one of two senior psychiatric residents, or a clinically experienced bachelor's-level research assistant. All four diagnosticians had been trained in the administration and scoring of these diagnostic instruments by the senior author, and adequate levels of interrater reliability had been obtained during this training period.

The following instruments were adminstered to each patient blind to his or her clinical diagnosis: 1) the Structured Clinical Interview for DSM-III-R Axis I Disorders (with a posttraumatic stress disorder module included that was devised at McLean) (Spitzer et al. 1990); 2) the DIB-R, a semistructured interview that can reliably distinguish clinically diagnosed borderline patients from those with other Axis II disorders (Zanarini et al. 1989b); and 3) the Revised Diagnostic Interview for Personality Disorders, a semistructured interview that reliably assesses the presence of the 13 Axis II disorders described in DSM-III-R (Zanarini et al. 1987b).

## Results

Eighty-seven patients met both the DIB-R and the DSM-III-R criteria for BPD, and 49 met the DSM-III-R criteria for at least one other type of nonborderline Axis II disorder. Borderline patients were similar to control subjects in their average age (30.3 ± 9.4 vs. 32.7 ± 9.4) and socioeconomic background, as measured by the five-point Hollingshead-Redlich Scale (Hollingshead 1957) (3.2 ± 1.1 vs. 2.9 ± 1.2). However, they were significantly more likely to be female than were control subjects (71.3% vs. 44.9%).

The lifetime prevalences of the disorders we have defined as compulsive and impulsive spectrum disorders are detailed in Table 2–2. As can be seen, 20.7% of our borderline cohort met the DSM-III-R criteria for OCD, 9.2% met the criteria for hypochondriasis, 8.1% met the criteria for "pure" anorexia nervosa, and 29.9% met the criteria for obsessive-compulsive personality disorder. As can also be seen, 72.4% of our borderline cohort met the DSM-III-R criteria for psychoactive substance use disorders. In addition, 32.2% met the DSM-III-R criteria for "pure" bulimia nervosa (20.7%) or mixed anorexia/bulimia nervosa (11.5%), and 25.3% met the criteria for antisocial personality disorder. None of these Axis I or Axis II disorders was significantly more common among our borderline patients than among the control subjects with personality disorders.

**Table 2–2.**    Lifetime prevalences of compulsive and impulsive
spectrum disorders

|  | BPD (%) | Other PD (%) |
|---|---|---|
| Obsessive-compulsive disorder | 20.7 | 12.2 |
| Hypochondriasis | 9.2 | 0.0 |
| Anorexia nervosa | 8.1 | 10.2 |
| Obsessive-compulsive personality disorder | 29.9 | 22.4 |
| Substance abuse | 72.4 | 67.3 |
| Other eating disorder | 32.2 | 20.4 |
| Antisocial personality disorder | 25.3 | 28.6 |

*Note.*   BPD = borderline personality disorder; PD = personality disorder.

The subsyndromal phenomenology of both a compulsive and an impulsive type that seems emblematic of the compulsive and impulsive features or aspects of BPD is detailed in Table 2–3. Most of the DSM-III-R criteria for obsessive-compulsive personality disorder were relatively common among our patients with BPD. Only lack of generosity was not reported by about one-quarter or more of our borderline sample. However, only one criterion of obsessive-compulsive personality disorder—indecisiveness—was reported by a significantly higher percentage of borderline patients than control subjects. As can also be seen, recent patterns (within the 2 years before the interview) of deliberate self-mutilation and suicidality were both very common among borderline patients and significantly more common among borderline patients than among control subjects with other Axis II personality disorders. Overall, 44.8% of our borderline patients met the DSM-III-R criteria for at least one compulsive spectrum disorder, and 83.9% met the DSM-III-R criteria for at least one impulsive spectrum disorder.

## Discussion

Five models of the relationship between Axis I and Axis II disorders have been proposed. Models I, II, and III have recently been re-

**Table 2–3.** Compulsive and impulsive symptomatology

|  | BPD (%) | Other PD (%) |
|---|---|---|
| Restricted expression of affection | 24.1 | 22.4 |
| Lack of generosity | 10.3 | 6.1 |
| Inability to discard worn-out objects | 34.5 | 20.4 |
| Extreme perfectionism | 43.7 | 34.7 |
| Preoccupation with details | 37.9 | 26.5 |
| Indecisiveness | 58.6 | 30.6** |
| Unreasonable insistence on own way | 52.9 | 44.9 |
| Overconscientiousness | 42.5 | 38.8 |
| Excessive devotion to work | 24.1 | 42.9* |
| Deliberate self-mutilation | 74.7 | 20.4*** |
| Suicide threats/gestures/attempts | 81.6 | 40.8*** |

*Note.* BPD = borderline personality disorder; PD = personality disorder.
*$P < .05$, **$P < .01$, ***$P < .001$ (corrected chi-square analyses).

viewed by Stein and colleagues (1993). Model I suggests that Axis I disorders arise as symptom clusters from the foundation of character pathology. Model II suggests that the presence of an Axis I disorder gives rise to the formation of maladaptive character traits and a level of functioning characteristic of a personality disorder. Model III suggests that some Axis I and Axis II disorders share a biochemical substrate that, in part, explains the overall picture of psychopathology with which the patient presents. The dimensional models of compulsivity–impulsivity proposed by Hollander and colleagues (Hollander 1993; Stein and Hollander 1993) and McElroy and colleagues (1992, 1993) are somewhat akin to Model III, in that they both suggest that a wide variety of seemingly disparate psychopathology can result, at least in part, from a common biochemical substrate.

Both Models IV and V seem more specific to BPD. Model IV, which arose from the work of van der Kolk and colleagues (van der Kolk and Greenberg 1987), suggests that severe childhood trauma alters a person's neurochemistry in such a way that he or she feels constantly hyperaroused and/or numb and that this alternation in a person's neurochemistry and sense of self will influence personality development in expectable, if maladaptive, ways. Model V, which we believe best captures the complexity of borderline psychopathology, is multifactorial in nature (Zanarini and Frankenburg 1994). It suggests that borderline symptomatology and its comorbid manifestations are the final end product of a complex admixture of innate temperament, difficult childhood experiences, and relatively subtle forms of neurological and biochemical dysfunction (which may be sequelae of these childhood experiences or innate vulnerabilities). It also suggests that there may be subgroups of borderline patients because of differing combinations and/or interactions of these various risk factors.

Most of the nine studies of the phenomenology of BPD reviewed in the previous section of this chapter reveal only a modest relationship between BPD and compulsive spectrum disorders. They also tend to reveal a strong relationship between BPD and what we have defined as impulse spectrum disorders.

In our most recent study of the phenomenology of BPD, we found high levels of impulse spectrum disorders that were similar to those found in most previous studies, including that by our own group. We also found a much stronger relationship between BPD and compulsive spectrum disorders than in most previous studies, including our own previous study of the phenomenology of BPD.

Some of these differences in prevalence rates of comorbid compulsive spectrum disorders may be due to differences in the DSM-III and DSM-III-R criteria sets for certain disorders. This may be particularly true for compulsive personality disorder (DSM-III) and obsessive-compulsive personality disorder (DSM-III-R): the former requires that the patient meet four of five criteria, whereas the latter requires that the patient meet five of nine criteria.

Some of these differences in comorbidity rates may also be due to differences in diagnostic methods. In general, it has been found that chart review studies yield the lowest rates, research interview–based studies yield the highest rates, and studies with a combination of clinical and research data yield intermediate rates (Zanarini et al. 1989a). This observation helps to explain the differences between our recent research interview–based study and the studies of Pope and colleagues (1983) and Frances and associates (1984), which used, respectively, chart reviews and clinical interviews to assess comorbidity. However, it does little to explain the differences in compulsive spectrum comorbidity found in our recent study and in our previous study, both of which used semistructured interviews to assess Axis I and Axis II phenomenology.

Perhaps the most parsimonious explanation is that our previous study was completed a decade ago and dealt with outpatients (many of whom, however, had been hospitalized previously), whereas our more recent study was completed about 3 years ago and dealt with acutely ill inpatients. It may be that this difference in treatment status and the much greater severity of illness of inpatients in the last several years have led to a difference in some of the comorbid disorders found in these otherwise similar borderline samples.

Clinicians have long recognized that borderline patients present with a complex admixture of compulsive symptoms, such as extreme perfectionism and the felt need to control some of the actions of others, and impulsive symptoms, such as temper outbursts and suicide threats. However, clinicians have also long recognized that some prototypic features of BPD, such as a pattern of self-mutilation, are a mixture of both compulsive and impulsive features. More specifically, some patients may feel driven to harm themselves and derive only minimal relief from doing so. Conversely, many patients hurt themselves impulsively in the middle of an interpersonal struggle and then feel substantially better after making their subjective pain tangible.

Several vignettes best illustrate this diversity of clinical presentations:

■ Vignette 1

Ms. A. is a 27-year-old single woman who first received psychiatric care at the age of 8. She has consistently been a shy, reserved, extremely fearful person. She has also consistently shown a strong desire to do the "right" thing and to do it perfectly, frequently asking for guidance and reassurance. As an adolescent, she frequently acted in an impulsive manner, having temper outbursts, breaking furniture, and cutting herself. As a young adult, she has shown both an obsessional character style and frank symptoms of OCD. Some of these symptoms relate to compulsive efforts to hide her feelings, and some relate to an obsessional preoccupation with suicide and the need to hurt herself.

■ Vignette 2

Ms. B. is a 20-year-old single woman who first received psychiatric care at the age of 18. She was an exceptional student and athlete, with a strong perfectionistic streak. Ms. B. developed a serious eating disorder in high school. Shortly after, she began making suicide attempts and cutting herself. She also began to abuse drugs, became sexually promiscuous, and repeatedly assaulted various family members. Her close relationships were extremely stormy, with frequent verbal outbursts and rageful attacks. Even when contained in the hospital, she often acted impulsively, frequently ending up in locked-door seclusion and restraints. However, at times, she also was troubled by obsessional thoughts about her self-worth and right to be alive.

The first vignette describes a basically obsessional patient who went through a circumscribed period of impulsivity. The second vignette describes an extremely impulsive patient who was a dutiful, obsessional child who still, later, occasionally displayed obsessional character traits. Both vignettes illustrate that patients with BPD tend to have both compulsive and impulsive personality features. Both vignettes also illustrate that the strength of these features may vary over time and may be related to both the maturational process and the presence of a comorbid disorder, such as substance abuse or OCD, that may strengthen the natural tendency toward impulsivity or compulsivity.

Our recent research results are consistent with this complex clinical view of borderline psychopathology. Our borderline sample showed high rates of both obsessional character traits and deliberate self-harm and suicidality. Our borderline sample also showed both suprisingly high rates of compulsive spectrum comorbidity and expectably high rates of impulsive spectrum comorbidity.

In terms of heuristic models, we believe that our results are most consistent with Model V (which subsumes Models III and IV), discussed earlier in this section. More specifically, recent research on temperament has found that a diagnosis of BPD (alone among Axis II disorders) is significantly associated with high levels of both harm avoidance (compulsivity) and novelty seeking (impulsivity) (Svrakic et al. 1993). In addition, recent studies have confirmed the results of earlier studies that found that a significantly high percentage of borderline patients report a childhood history of numerous forms of abuse (and neglect) (Paris et al. 1994; Zanarini et al. 1993).

Recent studies have also found that subtle forms of neurological and biochemical dysfunction are common in patients with BPD. More specifically, a series of studies have found that borderline patients often suffer from difficult-to-diagnose forms of neurological dysfunction (see Zanarini et al. 1994 for a review of studies in this area). In addition, biochemical studies have typically found low levels of serotonin in patients with problematic impulsivity, including patients with criteria-defined BPD (Coccaro et al. 1989; Hollander et al. 1994). A series of studies have also found that fluoxetine, a selective serotonin reuptake inhibitor, is effective in decreasing some types of impulsivity in borderline patients (Coccaro et al. 1990; Cornelius et al. 1991; Markovitz et al. 1991; Salzman 1993). However, elevated levels of serotonin have been found in many patients with OCD (Hollander et al. 1992; Insel et al. 1985), and fluoxetine (as well as other serotonergic agents) has also been found to be helpful in the treatment of this disorder (Hollander et al. 1991; Liebowitz et al. 1989).

Our study has found that patients with BPD often meet the criteria for both compulsive and impulsive spectrum disorders and that a high percentage report having both compulsive personality traits and high levels of pathognomonic impulsive behavioral patterns. It may be that borderline patients have particularly unstable serotonergic system functioning and that fluoxetine serves to alleviate both compulsive and impulsive symptoms in these (and other) patients by stabilizing the functioning of this neurotransmitter system (Hollander 1993). It may also be that other neurotransmitter systems (e.g., noradrenergic) are involved in mediating these behaviors and that interactions between these systems need to be explored.

In any case, further research is needed to assess whether less acutely disturbed borderline patients exhibit the same complicated pattern of comorbidity. Further research is also needed to assess the treatment implications of finding that borderline patients can exhibit symptomatology that spans the range of compulsive and impulsive psychopathology.

# References

Akiskal HS: Subaffective disorders: dysthymic, cyclothymic and bipolar II disorders in the "borderline" realm. Psychiatr Clin North Am 4:25–46, 1981

American Psychiatric Association: Diagnostic and Statistical Manual of Mental Disorders, 3rd Edition. Washington, DC, American Psychiatric Association, 1980

American Psychiatric Association: Diagnostic and Statistical Manual of Mental Disorders, 3rd Edition, Revised. Washington, DC, American Psychiatric Association, 1987

Andrulonis PA, Vogel NG: Comparison of borderline personality subcategories to schizophrenic and affective disorders. Br J Psychiatry 144:358–363, 1984

Baer L, Jenike MA: Personality disorders in obsessive-compulsive disorder, in Obsessive-Compulsive Disorders: Theory and Management. Edited by Jenike MA, Baer L, Minichiello WE. Chicago, IL, Year Book Medical, 1990, pp 76–88

Coccaro EF, Siever LJ, Klar HM, et al: Serotonergic studies in patients with affective and personality disorders: correlations with suicidal and impulsive aggressive behavior. Arch Gen Psychiatry 46:587–599, 1989

Coccaro EF, Astill JL, Herbert JL, et al: Fluoxetine treatment of impulsive aggression in DSM-III-R personality disorder patients. J Clin Psychopharmacol 10:373–375, 1990

Coid JW: An affective syndrome in psychopaths with borderline personality disorder. Br J Psychiatry 162:641–650, 1993

Cornelius JR, Soloff PH, Perel JM, et al: A preliminary trial of fluoxetine in refractory borderline patients. J Clin Psychopharmacol 11: 116–120, 1991

Endicott J, Spitzer RL: A diagnostic interview: the Schedule for Affective Disorders and Schizophrenia. Arch Gen Psychiatry 35:837–844, 1978

Frances A, Clarkin JF, Gilmore M, et al: Reliability of criteria for borderline personality disorder: a comparison of DSM-III and the Diagnostic Interview for Borderline Patients. Am J Psychiatry 141:1080–1084, 1984

Gunderson JG: Borderline Personality Disorder. Washington, DC, American Psychiatric Press, 1984

Gunderson JG, Kolb JE: Discriminating features of borderline patients. Am J Psychiatry 135:792–796, 1978

Gunderson JG, Singer MT: Defining borderline patients: an overview. Am J Psychiatry 132:1–10, 1975

Gunderson JG, Kolb JE, Austin V: The Diagnostic Interview for Borderlines. Am J Psychiatry 138:896–903, 1981

Herman JL, Perry JC, van der Kolk BA: Childhood trauma in borderline personality disorder. Am J Psychiatry 146:490–495, 1989

Hollander E: Introduction, in Obsessive-Compulsive–Related Disorders. Edited by Hollander E. Washington, DC, American Psychiatric Press, 1993, pp 1–16

Hollander E, DeCaria CM, Gully R, et al: Effects of chronic fluoxetine treatment on behavioral and neuroendocrine response to meta-chlorophenylpiperazine in obsessive-compulsive disorder. Psychiatry Res 36:1–17, 1991

Hollander E, DeCaria CM, Nitescu A, et al: Serotonergic function in obsessive-compulsive disorder: behavioral and neuroendocrine responses to oral m-chlorophenylpiperazine and fenfluramine in patients and healthy volunteers. Arch Gen Psychiatry 49:21–28, 1992

Hollander E, Stein DJ, DeCaria CM, et al: Serotonergic sensitivity in borderline personality disorder: preliminary findings. Am J Psychiatry 151:277–280, 1994

Hollingshead AB: Two Factor Index of Social Position. New Haven, CT, Department of Sociology, Yale University, 1957

Insel TR, Mueller EA, Alterman I, et al: Obsessive-compulsive disorder and serotonin: is there a connection? Biol Psychiatry 20:1174–1188, 1985

Jenike MA: Illness related to obsessive-compulsive disorder, in Obsessive-Compulsive Disorders: Theory and Management. Edited by Jenike MA, Baer L, Minichiello WE. Chicago, IL, Year Book Medical, 1990, pp 39–60

Kernberg OF: Borderline Conditions and Pathological Narcissism. New York, Jason Aronson, 1975

Liebowitz MR, Hollander E, Schneier F, et al: Fluoxetine treatment of obsessive-compulsive disorder: an open clinical trial. J Clin Psychopharmacol 9:423–427, 1989

Links PS, Steiner M, Offord DR, et al: Characteristics of borderline personality disorder: a Canadian study. Can J Psychiatry 33:336–340, 1988

Markovitz PJ, Calabrese JR, Schulz SC, et al: Fluoxetine in the treatment of borderline and schizotypal personality disorders. Am J Psychiatry 148:1064–1067, 1991

McElroy SL, Hudson JI Jr, Pope HG Jr, et al: The DSM-III-R impulse control disorders not elsewhere classified: clinical characteristics and relationship to other psychiatric disorders. Am J Psychiatry 149:318–327, 1992

McElroy SL, Hudson JI Jr, Phillips KA, et al: Clinical and theoretical implications of a possible link between obsessive-compulsive and impulse control disorders. Depression 1:121–132, 1993

McGlashan TH: The borderline syndrome, II: is it a variant of schizophrenia or affective disorder? Arch Gen Psychiatry 40:1319–1323, 1983

McGlashan TH, Heinssen RK: Narcissistic, antisocial, and noncomorbid subgroups of borderline disorder: are they distinct entities by long-term clinical profile? Psychiatr Clin North Am 12:653–670, 1989

Ogata SN, Silk KR, Goodrich S, et al: Childhood sexual and physical abuse in adult patients with borderline personality disorder. Am J Psychiatry 147:1008–1013, 1990

Oldham JM, Skodol AE, Kellman HD, et al: Diagnosis of DSM-III-R personality disorders by two structured interviews: patterns of comorbidity. Am J Psychiatry 149:213–220, 1992

Paris J, Zweig-Frank H, Guzder J: Psychological risk factors for borderline personality disorder in female patients. Compr Psychiatry 35:301–305, 1994

Perry JC, Cooper SH: Psychodynamics, symptoms, and outcome in borderline and antisocial personality disorders and bipolar type II affective disorder, in The Borderline: Current Empirical Research. Edited by McGlashan TH. Washington, DC, American Psychiatric Press, 1985, pp 19–41

Pope HG Jr, Jonas JM, Hudson JI Jr, et al: The validity of DSM-III borderline personality disorder. Arch Gen Psychiatry 40:23–30, 1983

Robins LN, Helzer JE, Croughan J, et al: National Institute of Mental Health Diagnostic Interview Schedule: its history, characteristics, and validity. Arch Gen Psychiatry 38:381–389, 1981

Salzman C: Effect of fluoxetine on anger in borderline personality disorder. Paper presented at the Third International Congress on the Disorders of Personality, Cambridge, MA, September 1993

Shearer SL, Peters CP, Quaytman MS, et al: Frequency and correlates of childhood sexual and physical abuse histories in adult female borderline inpatients. Am J Psychiatry 147:214–216, 1990

Skodol AE, Oldham JM, Hyler SE, et al: Fears and inhibitions: patterns of comorbidity. Paper presented at the 146th annual meeting of the American Psychiatric Association, Philadelphia, PA, May 1994

Spitzer RL, Williams JBW: Structured Clinical Interview for DSM-III Axis II Disorders. New York, New York State Psychiatric Institute, 1983

Spitzer RL, Williams JBW: Structured Clinical Interview for DSM-III Axis I Disorders. New York, New York State Psychiatric Institute, 1984

Spitzer RL, Endicott J, Robins E: Research Diagnostic Criteria: rationale and reliability. Arch Gen Psychiatry 35:773–779, 1978

Spitzer RL, Williams JBW, Gibbon M, et al: Structured Clinical Interview for DSM-III-R Axis I Disorders. Washington, DC, American Psychiatric Press, 1990

Stein DJ, Hollander E: The spectrum of obsessive-compulsive–related disorders, in Obsessive-Compulsive–Related Disorders. Edited by Hollander E. Washington, DC, American Psychiatric Press, 1993, pp 241–271

Stein DJ, Hollander E, Skodol AE: Anxiety disorders and personality disorders: a review. Journal of Personality Disorders 7:87–104, 1993

Stern A: Psychoanalytic investigation of and therapy in the borderline group of neuroses. Psychoanal Q 7:467–489, 1938

Stone MH: The Borderline Syndromes: Constitution, Personality, and Adaptation. New York, McGraw-Hill, 1980

Svrakic DM, Whitehead C, Przybeck TR, et al: Differential diagnosis of personality disorders by the seven-factor model of temperament and character. Arch Gen Psychiatry 50:991–999, 1993

van der Kolk BA, Greenberg MS: The psychobiology of the trauma response: developmental issues in the psychobiology of attachment and separation, in van der Kolk BA: Psychological Trauma. Washington, DC, American Psychiatric Press, 1987, pp 63–87

Wender PH: The contribution of the adoption studies to an understanding of the phenomenology and etiology of borderline schizophrenia, in Borderline Personality Disorders: The Concept, the Syndrome, the Patient. Edited by Hartocollis P. New York, International Universities Press, 1977, pp 255–269

Westen D, Ludolph P, Misle B, et al: Physical and sexual abuse in adolescent girls with borderline personality disorder. Am J Orthopsychiatry 60:55–66, 1990

Zanarini MC: BPD as an impulse spectrum disorder, in Borderline Personality Disorder: Etiology and Treatment. Edited by Paris J. Washington, DC, American Psychiatric Press, 1993, pp 67–85

Zanarini MC, Frankenburg FR: Emotional hypochondriasis, hyperbole, and the borderline patient. Journal of Psychotherapy Practice and Research 3:25–36, 1994

Zanarini MC, Frankenburg FR, Chauncey DL, et al: The Diagnostic Interview for Personality Disorders: interrater and test-retest reliability. Compr Psychiatry 28:467–480, 1987a

Zanarini MC, Frankenburg FR, Chauncey DL: The Revised Diagnostic Interview for Personality Disorders. Belmont, MA, McLean Hospital, Psychosocial Research Program, 1987b

Zanarini MC, Gunderson JG, Frankenburg FR: Axis II phenomenology of borderline personality disorder. Paper presented at the World Psychiatric Association Regional Symposium, Washington, DC, October 1988

Zanarini MC, Gunderson JG, Frankenburg FR: Axis I phenomenology of borderline personality disorder. Compr Psychiatry 30:149–156, 1989a

Zanarini MC, Gunderson JG, Frankenburg FR, et al: The Revised Diagnostic Interview for Borderlines: discriminating BPD from other Axis II disorders. Journal of Personality Disorders 3:10–18, 1989b

Zanarini MC, Gunderson JG, Marino MF, et al: Childhood experiences of borderline patients. Compr Psychiatry 30:18–25, 1989c

Zanarini MC, Dubo ED, Lewis RE, et al: Childhood factors associated with the development of borderline personality disorder. Paper presented at the Third International Congress on the Disorders of Personality, Cambridge, MA, September 1993

Zanarini MC, Kimble CR, Williams AA: Neurological dysfunction in borderline patients and Axis II control subjects, in Biological and Neurobehavioral Studies of Borderline Personality Disorder. Edited by Silk KR. Washington, DC, American Psychiatric Press, 1994, pp 159–175

# 3

# Assessment of the Impulsive-Compulsive Spectrum of Behavior by the Seven-Factor Model of Temperament and Character

### C. Robert Cloninger, M.D.

Impulsivity and compulsivity have been described in many different ways because of uncertainty about the psychobiological taxonomy of personality. The number and content of the disorders

Supported in part by grants from the National Institute of Mental Health (MH-31302, MH-46276, MH-46280) and the National Institute on Alcohol Abuse and Alcoholism (AA-08028 and AA-08401).

All tables in this chapter have been adapted, with permission, from Cloninger CR, Przybeck TR, Svrakic DM, et al.: *The Temperament and Character Inventory (TCI): A Guide to Its Development and Use*. St. Louis, MO, Washington University Center for the Psychobiology of Personality, 1994.

and dimensions of personality related to impulsive and compulsive behavior have remained in question because of the apparent absence of any definitive criterion—or "gold standard"—to specify the fundamental causes of behavioral variation. Neither clinical nor neurobiological strategies permit resolution of a unique way to specify the causal structure of impulsive and compulsive behavior. This ambiguity persists because there are always an infinite number of alternative ways to explain the correlations among clinical symptoms and neurobiological signs in groups of unrelated individuals. Fortunately, studies of genetic architecture in groups of related individuals do provide a unique criterion for the underlying causal structure of personality, including impulsive and compulsive behavior.

Kendell (1982) disparaged the proliferation of partly overlapping sets of diagnostic criteria in psychiatry and offered some statistical criteria for "cutting nature at its joints." For example, he suggested that discrete disorders could be recognized by evidence of bimodality in the distribution of symptoms that discriminate different groups of patients. Although there has been some success with this to distinguish heterogeneous psychoses (Cloninger et al. 1985), there is little evidence for discrete categories or disease entities in the personality realm.

Likewise, many alternative quantitative measures of personality have been advocated, but no consensus about the number or content of their dimensions has been reached (John 1990). Such quantitative variation is prominent in both clinical and neurobiological variation related to personality traits. Although much is known about brain structure and function, there is no consensus about its functional organization (Carroll and Barrett 1991). Alternative models of the organization of brain systems underlying personality remain controversial when they are based on neurobiological and clinical findings about groups of individuals. Experimental neurobiological studies can establish particular causal connections (Adamec 1991) but cannot provide an overall model of the number or content of dimensions underlying personality. Likewise, descriptive information about clinical variation in groups of individuals cannot provide a unique model of impulsive and compulsive behavior because of the indeterminacy of factor-analytic and clustering techniques.

In contrast, knowledge of the mechanisms of genetic and environmental resemblance within families is sufficiently strong that the causal architecture of traits purported to measure impulsivity and other personality traits can be directly assessed. For traits that are only moderately heritable, such as impulsivity, large samples of twins provide sufficient power to specify the underlying architecture (Heath et al. 1994). Such studies have now been conducted in Australia and the United States with measures of personality and provide a unique and specific model of the causal components of impulsivity and compulsivity.

In this chapter I first describe the early stages of testing and revision from 1986 to the present that were designed to address questions about the impulsive-compulsive spectrum of behavior. I then describe the model of temperament that recent twin studies have confirmed to correspond well with the unique genetic structure of personality. According to this model, impulsive behavior is related to four heritable temperament traits: high novelty seeking, low harm avoidance, low persistence, and, rarely, low reward dependence. In contrast, compulsive behavior is related to the converse profile: low novelty seeking, high harm avoidance, high persistence, and, rarely, high reward dependence. After describing the model, I summarize available applications of this model to impulsive and compulsive behavior in samples from the general population and from treatment settings.

# Development of the Temperament Model

I began work on the structure of personality to develop a general model to explain the differences between patients with somatization disorder (Briquet's syndrome) and generalized anxiety disorder (Cloninger 1986). I observed that patients with somatic anxiety had impulsive-aggressive personality traits, whereas those with generalized cognitive anxiety had obsessive-compulsive personality traits. Hysteric persons and others with somatic anxiety had been described by Eysenck as "neurotic extraverts," whereas neurotic persons with cognitive anxiety had been described as "neurotic introverts" by use of the Eysenck Personality Questionnaire (EPQ; Eysenck and Eysenck 1976) and its forerunners.

I sought a general model that would apply to both normal and abnormal personality, as did the model of Eysenck, but observed that Eysenck's model was unacceptable. The dimensions of Neuroticism and Extraversion had been specified on the basis of factor analyses of the phenotypic (observed) structure of personality. Phenotypic variation is the product of the interaction of both genetic and environmental factors, and Eysenck assumed that the phenotypic and genotypic structures were the same. This is equivalent to assuming that genetic and environmental factors influence behavior in the same way. However, this assumption was questionable. In particular, it was already known that extraversion was genetically heterogeneous (Eaves and Eysenck 1975). It is composed of two factors that are largely genetically independent—impulsivity and sociability—and appears to be a single behavioral dimension because of shared environmental influences. In other words, genetic and environmental influences do not influence behavior in the same way, contrary to Eysenck's assumption. In addition, Gray (1981) had shown that anti-anxiety drugs affected both neuroticism (decreases) and extraversion (increases), suggesting that "anxiety" was more parsimoniously defined by a single dimension combining the two, that is, by a dimension corresponding to neurotic introvert. Likewise, "impulsivity" was defined as a dimension independent of anxiety, that is, by neurotic extravert. In addition, he showed that the rate of operant learning in response to signals of punishment was maximal along the "anxiety," or compulsivity, dimension, not the dimension represented by Eysenck's neuroticism factor. The rate of operant learning in response to signals of reward was maximal along the "impulsivity" dimension, not Eysenck's extraversion factor.

Two dimensions are too few to provide a comprehensive model of personality. However, Eysenck's psychoticism dimension was shown to be genetically heterogeneous, so it was an unsatisfactory scale to measure a third dimension of heritable personality traits (Heath and Martin 1990). Fortunately, the Swedish psychiatrist Henrik Sjobring had described a model of personality in terms of its underlying neurogenetic basis that provided clues to the content of a third dimension. Sjobring (1973) called his three dimensions *solidity* (vs. impulsive), *validity* (vs. compulsive), and *stability* (vs. moody sociability). He modeled the description of the low variants of these three on impulsive hysteric persons, compulsive psychasthenic persons, and sociable depressive persons, respectively. Measures from the Karolinska Scales of Personality (KSP; Schalling and Edman 1986) related to low solidity (impulsivity) and low validity (anxious compulsivity) had been related to somatic and anticipatory anxiety, respectively (Schalling et al. 1973; Schalling and Edman 1986). Therefore, Sjobring's description of stability provided a tentative construct for a third heritable dimension of temperament.

Because of the ambiguity of such descriptive adjectives, I developed a neurobiological learning model to guide the rational description of personality assessment instruments (Cloninger 1987a, 1987b, 1991). Initially, I hypothesized that the temperament systems in the brain were functionally organized as independently varying systems for the activation, maintenance, and inhibition of behavior in response to specific classes of stimuli. Behavioral activation involved the activation of behavior in response to novelty and signals of reward or relief of punishment; accordingly, individual differences in such activatability were called *novelty seeking*. Behavioral inhibition occurred in response to signals of punishment or nonreward, so individual differences in inhibitability were called *harm avoidance*. Behavior that was previously rewarded was later maintained for a while without continued reinforcement, and individual differences in such maintenance was called *reward dependence*. Reward dependence initially included the sociability and persistence described by Sjobring as aspects of low stability. However, recent work has shown that dependence on warm social attachments and persistence, despite intermittent reinforcement, are usually dissociated and are independently inherited (Cloninger et al. 1993).

The Tridimensional Personality Questionnaire (TPQ; Cloninger 1987b) was developed to test these hypotheses and to evaluate their adequacy as a general model of personality. Each of the three major dimensions has four subscales, including persistence as one subscale of reward dependence. Confirmatory factor analysis supported the proposed factor structure with persistence as a fourth dimension (Cloninger et al. 1991; Nixon and Parsons 1989; Waller et al. 1991). In both normal and abnormal samples, the putative dimensions were highly reliable and stable despite mood state; only harm avoidance was transiently increased when individuals were agitated or depressed (Brown et al. 1992; Cloninger 1987b; Cloninger et al. 1991; Joffe et al. 1993; Perna et al. 1992; Svrakic et al. 1992), and novelty seeking may be transiently increased when bipolar patients are subclinically hypomanic (Strakowski et al. 1993). The structure and stability of temperament have been replicated in several different cultures with translations of the TPQ: the Czech Republic (Kozeny et al. 1989), the former Yugoslavia (Svrakic et al. 1991), Japan (Takeuchi et al. 1993), Italy (Perna et al. 1992), and Norway (Strandbygaard and Jensen 1992), among others.

Most importantly, recent large-scale twin studies have confirmed that the four temperaments of novelty seeking, harm avoidance, reward dependence (now limited to social sensitivity), and persistence are genetically homogeneous and independent of one another (Heath et al. 1994; Stallings et al., in press). These twin studies have shown that there are environmental influences that sometimes induce a weak correlation between persistence and reward dependence but no shared genetic factors (Stallings et al., in press). Alternative models of personality comprise genetically heterogeneous factors.

It is remarkable that the *four-factor model of temperament* can, in retrospect, be seen as a four-dimensional interpretation of the ancient four temperaments: individuals differ in the degree to which they are melancholic (comparable to harm avoidance), choleric (comparable to novelty seeking), sanguine (comparable to reward dependence), and phlegmatic (comparable to persistence). However, now the four temperaments are genetically independent dimensions that occur in all factorial combinations, rather than mutually exclusive categories.

# Development of the Character Model

The model of four temperaments provided an excellent description of traditional subtypes of personality disorder (Cloninger 1987b) but proved unable to distinguish whether someone had any personality disorder (Cloninger et al. 1993). Fortunately, studies comparing the TPQ to other personality inventories helped to identify additional aspects of personality that were not accounted for by its temperament dimensions. These included measures of mature self-directed behavior, cooperativeness, and self-transcendence, as summarized in Table 3–1 (Cloninger et al. 1993).

The characterological aspects of personality involve individual differences in self-concepts about goals and values, in contrast to the temperaments, which involve differences in automatic emotional reactions and habits. Such self-concepts modify the significance or meaning of what is experienced, thereby also changing

**Table 3–1.**    Descriptors of individuals who score high and low on the three character dimensions

| Character dimension | Descriptors of extreme variants | |
|---|---|---|
|  | High | Low |
| Self-directedness | Responsible | Blaming |
|  | Purposeful | Goal-less |
|  | Resourceful | Passive |
|  | Self-accepting | Wishful |
|  | Disciplined | Undisciplined |
| Cooperative | Tender-hearted | Intolerant |
|  | Empathic | Insensitive |
|  | Helpful | Selfish |
|  | Compassionate | Revengeful |
|  | Principled | Opportunistic |
| Self-transcendent | Self-forgetful | Unimaginative |
|  | Transpersonal | Controlling |
|  | Spiritual | Materialistic |
|  | Enlightened | Possessive |
|  | Idealistic | Conventional |

emotional reactions. Accordingly, individuals with the same temperament may behave differently as a result of differences in character development. For example, an individual high in novelty seeking and low in harm avoidance may have an impulsive personality disorder if he or she is low in self-directedness and cooperativeness, or the person may be a mature and daring explorer, inquisitive scientist, or acquisitive businessman. This indicates that clinical treatments directed at character development may prove to be promising. A comprehensive questionnaire for measuring all seven dimensions of personality, called the Temperament and Character Inventory (TCI), has been developed and is available for clinical and research use (Cloninger et al. 1993; Svrakic et al. 1993).

According to my psychobiological theory, *character development* involves changes in the propositional memory system, whereas *temperament* involves individual differences in procedural memory (Cloninger et al. 1993). Recent evidence regarding these cognitive and neurobiological differences in humans and other animals are reviewed elsewhere (Cloninger et al. 1994). Here, I summarize available clinical studies relevant to the impulsive and compulsive spectra of behavior.

## Relations of Alternative Models of Normal Personality

The major models of personality all include measures of impulsive and compulsive behavior, but despite the similarity in labels, these models overlap only partly with one another. Measures with the same name, such as impulsiveness, often measure different things. In this section I describe the relations among alternative measures of impulsivity/somatic anxiety and compulsivity/cognitive anxiety and relate these to the heritable dimensions of temperament.

The correlations among the TPQ temperament dimensions and the KSP (Schalling and Edman 1986) are presented in Table 3–2. The KSP, which was developed by Schalling with strong influences from Sjobring's ideas, provides measures of anxiety and impulsivity

**Table 3–2.**     Correlations (× 100) between Cloninger's Tridimensional Personality Questionnaire (TPQ) temperament dimensions and Schalling's Karolinska Scales of Personality (KSP) in a psychiatric outpatient sample ($N = 50$) and a general population sample ($N = 2,420$ women)

| KSP factors | Cloninger TPQ temperament dimensions | | | |
| | Harm avoidance | Novelty seeking | Reward dependence | Persistence |
|---|---|---|---|---|
| Psychic anxiety | 77*/67* | 4/–15 | 7/–6 | 30/13 |
| Somatic anxiety | 61*/53* | 8/2 | 2/0 | 37*/13 |
| Muscle tension | 51*/46* | 23/0 | 11/3 | 27/17 |
| | | | | |
| Monotony avoidance | –43*/–11 | 34*/28* | 30*/10 | 17/15 |
| Impulsivity | –13/1 | 67*/31* | 12/6 | 0/7 |

$*P < .05$.

*Source.*     Data for the psychiatric outpatient sample derived from Brown et al. 1992, and those for the general population sample derived from Stallings et al., in press.

corresponding to Gray's distinctions. The relations are similar both in clinical samples (Brown et al. 1992) and in a general population sample (Stallings et al., in press). Each of the KSP anxiety scales is highly correlated with harm avoidance. In contrast, KSP impulsivity is moderately to highly correlated with high novelty seeking. KSP monotony avoidance, like Eysenck's Extraversion, is a composite of low harm avoidance, high novelty seeking, and, possibly, high reward dependence.

Another informative way to consider the interrelations among mutiple measures of multiple traits is to carry out a joint factor analysis. The results of a joint analysis of Cloninger's TPQ, Schalling's KSP, and Eysenck's EPQ are summarized in Table 3–3. Four factors have eigenvalues greater than unity, and these correspond to the four TPQ temperaments. Factor 1 is specified by high TPQ harm avoidance, KSP psychic or cognitive anxiety, and EPQ neurotic introversion (i.e., low Extraversion and high Neuroticism).

**Table 3–3.**    Joint factor analysis of Tridimensional Personality
Questionnaire (TPQ), Eysenck Personality Questionnaire
(EPQ), and Karolinska Scales of Personality (KSP) scales
($N = 4,119$)

| | Oblique promax factor loadings ($\times$ 100) | | | |
|---|---|---|---|---|
| **Subscale** | **F1** | **F2** | **F3** | **F4** |
| KSP: Psychic anxiety | 78 | 29 | | |
| HA1: Anticipatory anxiety | 73 | | | |
| HA2: Fear of uncertainty | 69 | | | |
| HA3: Fear of strangers | 68 | | | |
| KSP: Somatic anxiety | 57 | 45 | | |
| EPQ: Neuroticism | 66 | | | |
| KSP: Muscle tension | 58 | 43 | | |
| HA4: Fatigability | 54 | | | |
| NS1: Exploratory | −32 | 25 | 28 | |
| EPQ: Extraversion | −44 | 34 | | 28 |
| | | | | |
| KSP: Monotony avoidance | | 70 | | |
| KSP: Impulsivity | | 57 | | |
| RD2: Persistence | | 33 | | |
| | | | | |
| NS2: Impulsiveness | | | 62 | |
| NS4: Disorderliness | | | 59 | |
| NS3: Extravagance | | | 50 | |
| EPQ: Lie (social conformity) | | | −39 | |
| | | | | |
| RD4: Dependence | | | | 56 |
| RD3: Attachment | | | | 51 |
| RD1: Sentimentality | | | | 34 |
| EPQ: Psychoticism | | | 28 | −38 |
| | | | | |
| Percentage variance explained | 19% | 8% | 7% | 5% |

*Note.*    Factor loadings < .25 omitted. F2 and F3 correlated +.39. HA = harm
avoidance; NS = novelty seeking; RD = reward dependence.
*Source.*    Data derived from Stallings et al., in press.

Factor 2 involves somatic anxiety, novelty seeking (the common denominator of KSP monotony avoidance and KSP impulsivity), and persistence. Factor 3 is defined by high TPQ novelty seeking and low EPQ Lie scores. Factor 4 is defined by high TPQ reward dependence and low EPQ psychoticism (i.e., toughmindedness). Thus, Eysenck's psychoticism does correspond partly to low reward dependence, even though the former is heterogeneous.

The results with the KSP indicate that impulsiveness and anxiety are both multidimensional phenomena. Anxiety has both cognitive (harm avoidance) and somatic (novelty seeking) components. Impulsivity comprises both high novelty seeking and low harm avoidance. This interpretation is further supported by comparison of the TPQ with components of Zuckerman's (1984) Sensation Seeking Scale and other measures of antisocial behavior and alcohol abuse (Table 3–4). In a sample of 298 college students, each of the subscales of sensation seeking were correlated moderately with high novelty seeking and low harm avoidance. Socialization, a reverse scored measure of delinquency and antisocial conduct from the California Psychological Inventory (Gough 1969), was correlated with low novelty seeking, high reward dependence, and high harm avoidance. Conversely, antisocial behavior, risk of alcohol abuse, and history of alcohol abuse had the opposite profile (high novelty seeking, low reward dependence, and low harm avoidance) in college students.

Likewise, in male veterans hospitalized for substance abuse, sensation seeking was moderately correlated with high novelty seeking (Table 3–5) and low harm avoidance (Table 3–6). In particular, thrill seeking on the Sensation Seeking Scale is highly correlated with low fear of uncertainty (HA2) and moderately correlated with exploratory excitability (NS1). Thus, sensation seeking is an etiologically complex process involving the interaction of multiple separately inherited temperament dimensions (Cloninger 1988).

Tellegen's Multidimensional Personality Questionnaire (MPQ) provides other measures of impulsive and compulsive behaviors (Cloninger 1987b; Waller et al. 1991). Tellegen developed 11 primary scales, which have three second-order dimensions of person-

**Table 3–4.**    Correlations of Tridimensional Personality
Questionnaire (TPQ) temperament dimensions and
sensation-seeking subscales, California Psychological
Inventory (CPI) socialization, and alcohol-related
variables in college students (*N* = 298)

| Variable | Correlations (× 100) with TPQ temperament dimensions | | |
| --- | --- | --- | --- |
| | Harm avoidance | Novelty seeking | Reward dependence |
| Sensation seeking | | | |
| Thrill seeking | −44* | 37* | −5 |
| Experience seeking | −23* | 31* | −5 |
| Disinhibition | −24* | 44* | −10 |
| Boredom susceptibility | −23* | 35* | −29* |
| CPI socialization | 17 | −32* | 28* |
| Risk of alcoholism (MacAndrews Scale) | −44* | 19* | −13 |
| Alcohol abuse history (MAST) | −7 | 18* | −5 |
| Current alcohol use | | | |
| Quantity | −13 | 40* | −11 |
| Frequency | −16 | 23* | −5 |

*Note.*    MAST = Michigan Alcohol Screening Test (Selzer 1971); MacAndrews
Scale (MacAndrews 1965).
*P < .05.
*Source.*    Data derived from Earleywine et al. 1992.

ality that he calls "positive emotionality" (like extraversion), "negative emotionality" (like neuroticism), and "constraint" (like compulsivity). An interbattery factor analysis in a general population sample gave the loadings of the MPQ on the four dimensions of the TPQ, as shown in Table 3–7 (Waller et al. 1991). High harm avoidance was correlated with high MPQ stress reactivity and low MPQ well-being. As with KSP impulsivity, MPQ impulsiveness (i.e., low constraint) was highly correlated with high novelty seeking. Likewise, high MPQ danger seeking (also called low MPQ harm avoidance) resembled KSP monotony avoidance in that it

**Table 3–5.** Standardized regression of novelty-seeking (NS) subscales on Sensation Seeking Scale subscales (*N* = 115 male inpatient veterans)

| Novelty-seeking subscale | Zuckerman's Sensation Seeking Scale components | | | |
| --- | --- | --- | --- | --- |
| | Thrill seeking | Experience seeking | Disinhibition | Boredom susceptibility |
| NS1 Exploratory | 33*** | 14 | 25** | 7 |
| NS2 Impulsive | −8 | 0 | −7 | 5 |
| NS3 Extravagant | 2 | 5 | 21* | 8 |
| NS4 Disorderly | 14 | 20 | 29** | 25 |

*Note.* Zero-order correlation sensation seeking and NS total scores = .43 ($P < .001$); set correlation $R = .58$***.
*$P < .05$; **$P < .01$; ***$P < .001$.
*Source.* Data derived from McCourt et al. 1993.

**Table 3–6.** Standardized regression of harm-avoidance (HA) subscales on Sensation Seeking Scale subscales (*N* = 115 male inpatients)

| Harm-avoidance subscale | Zuckerman's Sensation Seeking Scale components | | | |
| --- | --- | --- | --- | --- |
| | Thrill seeking | Experience seeking | Disinhibition | Boredom susceptibility |
| HA1 Pessimistic | 11 | 21 | 5 | 24* |
| HA2 Fearful | −61*** | −37*** | −23* | −27* |
| HA3 Shy | 14 | 18 | −5 | 12 |
| HA4 Fatigable | −5 | 8 | 4 | 2 |

*Note.* Set correlation $R = .61$***.
*$P < .05$; ***$P < .001$.
*Source.* Data derived from McCourt et al. 1993.

**Table 3–7.** Loadings (× 100) of primary factors of Tellegen's
Multidimensional Personality Questionnaire (MPQ) on
four-factor structure of the Tridimensional Personality
Questionnaire (TPQ) in a general population sample
(*N* = 1,236)

| MPQ factor | Harm avoidance | Novelty seeking | Reward dependence | Persistence |
|---|---|---|---|---|
| | **Cloninger TPQ temperament dimensions** | | | |
| Stress reaction | 74 | 2 | 8 | 28 |
| Well-being | −64 | 8 | 21 | −2 |
| Social potency | −56 | 33 | 7 | 26 |
| Danger seeking | −33 | 29 | −31 | 0 |
| Impulsiveness | 6 | 80 | −24 | −3 |
| Social closeness | −12 | 22 | 76 | 4 |
| Achievement | −34 | 17 | −9 | 76 |
| Alienation | 27 | 2 | −16 | 25 |
| Aggression | 4 | 22 | −24 | 2 |
| Absorption | −8 | 18 | 23 | 16 |

*Source.* Data derived from Waller et al. 1991.

was moderately correlated with low harm avoidance and high
novelty seeking. However, MPQ danger seeking was negatively
correlated with reward dependence, whereas KSP monotony
avoidance was positively correlated with reward dependence.
MPQ social closeness and achievement were closely related to
TPQ reward dependence and persistence, respectively. Three
primary MPQ scales—alienation, aggression, and absorption—
had no strong correlations with the TPQ temperament dimensions and partly guided the development of three corresponding
character scales.

The MPQ was largely derived from studies of healthy subjects
in Minnesota, whereas the Minnesota Multiphasic Personality Inventory (MMPI) was originally based on studies of clinical criterion
groups. Nevertheless, many scales can be derived from the MMPI

pool and have been validated in both psychiatrically healthy and psychiatrically ill samples. Analysis of the 12 TPQ subscales and the MMPI provided evidence that many of the TPQ subscales measure what they are described as measuring, at least for novelty seeking and harm avoidance, in which there is substantial overlap between the TPQ and MMPI (Wetzel et al. 1992) (Table 3–8). Analysis of the major factors derived from the MMPI by Welsh and Eichman revealed extensive close overlap with harm avoidance and its subscales. However, the MMPI measures reward dependence and persistence poorly, and the temperament dimensions of the TPQ do not measure the MMPI repression factor, which indicates difficulty coping maturely with societal demands. Later work has shown that low self-directedness and low cooperativeness are correlated with extensive use of immature defense mechanisms, including repression (R. T. Mulder, P. R. Joyce, J. D. Sellman, et al., unpublished data, 1994).

Other tests purporting to be comprehensive models of personality propose five to seven personality dimensions (Digman 1989; John 1990; Waller and Zavala 1993). Although the content of alternative five-factor models is variable (Zuckerman et al. 1993), the NEO–Personality Inventory (NEO-PI) has been shown to be stable in longitudinal studies (Costa and McCrae 1991). The NEO-PI "Big Five" factors include measures of extraversion and neuroticism, as in the EPQ, and measures of agreeability and conscientiousness, which overlap with the EPQ psychoticism and social conformity (Lie) scales. The content of the fifth factor is more controversial, varying from openness to intellect to culture. The relations among the TCI seven-factor model and the NEO five-factor model are shown in Table 3–9. The TCI measures both the four TPQ temperament dimensions and the three character dimensions described earlier. In brief, the NEO scales are correlated with multiple TCI dimensions. The NEO and TCI overlap extensively in a complex manner, and the five NEO factors explain much variability in five of the TCI dimensions. TCI persistence and self-transcendence are weakly explained by NEO measures. Interestingly, individual subscales of the TCI relate to individual NEO factors, so the TCI

**Table 3–8.**    Joint factor analysis of the Tridimensional Personality Questionnaire (TPQ) and the Minnesota Multiphasic Personality Inventory (MMPI) in a sample of psychiatric inpatients ($N = 88$)

| Personality scale | Varimax factor loadings ($\times$ 100) | | | |
|---|---|---|---|---|
| | F1 | F2 | F3 | F4 |
| MMPI Anxiety | | | | |
|   Welsh factor | 92 | | | |
|   Eichman factor | 86 | | | |
| MMPI Somatic concern | 68 | | | |
| TPQ Harm avoidance | 68 | 38 | | |
| MMPI Acting out impulses | 63 | −30 | | |
| MMPI Repression | | | | |
|   Welsh factor | | 88 | | |
|   Eichman factor | | 90 | | |
| TPQ Sentimentality (RD1) | | | 68 | |
| TPQ Attachment (RD3) | −38 | | 54 | |
| TPQ Dependence (RD4) | | | 64 | |
| TPQ Persistence (RD2) | | | 33 | −69 |
| TPQ Novelty seeking | | | | 84 |

*Note.*    RD = reward dependence.
*Source.*    Data derived from Wetzel et al. 1992.

can be used to estimate dimensions of both the five- and the seven-factor models.

In summary, joint analysis of the TPQ with alternative personality inventories provides strong support for four dimensions of temperament and three dimensions of character. These consistently emerge in joint analysis of multiple inventories, although only the TCI measures all seven dimensions in a strong and direct manner. The factor pattern was reproduced in both general and clinical populations by independent investigators (Bagby et al. 1992; Kleifield et al. 1993; Waller et al. 1991).

# Clinical Applications to Anxiety Disorders

According to the *biosocial learning theory of personality* (Cloninger 1986), individuals with various anxiety disorders are all expected to exhibit high levels of harm avoidance. The TPQ has been used to evaluate this prediction in several studies of anxiety disorders, the results of which are summarized in Table 3–10. Individuals with all types of anxiety disorders are high in harm avoidance and usually are in the top quintile of the general population. They are usually about average in novelty seeking, regardless of the subtype of anxiety disorder. Individuals with social phobia are also reported to be low in reward dependence, suggesting that social phobia involves both fear and low sociability, but this is based on a single study (M. E. Tancer and R. N. Golden, abstract for Society of Biological Psychiatry, written communication, 1993). In contrast, Pfohl and co-workers (1990) found patients with obsessive-compulsive disorder to be high in reward dependence, but this finding was not replicated in a second study (L. J. Summerfeldt, M. Richter, and R. M. Bagby, written communication, November 1993). Theoretically, the minority of obsessional patients who are high in both harm avoidance and persistence are expected to be most difficult to manage, but systematic treatment studies are not yet available.

# Differential Personality Profiles in Eating Disorders

Eating disorders constitute a valuable area for personality assessment because different subtypes are associated with impulsive versus compulsive patterns of motivated behavior. Bulimic patients alternately binge and purge so they are expected to have approach-avoidance conflicts, dysthymia, and borderline or histrionic personalities, all of which are associated with exhibiting high levels of both novelty seeking and harm avoidance. In contrast, restrictive anorexic patients have been described as obsessional personalities and are expected to exhibit high levels of harm avoidance and

**Table 3–9.** Correlations among seven Temperament and Character Inventory (TCI) dimensions and components of Eysenck's and Norman's models, along with descriptors that discriminate each significant factorial combination

| TCI factor | Surgent Extravert (Introvert) | Emotional Neurotic (Stable) | Agreeable Tender (Tough) | Conscience Conform (No lie) | Culture Open (Narrow) |
|---|---|---|---|---|---|
| **Temperament** | | | | | |
| Novelty seeking | 36 (45) Adventurous Impulsive Extravagant | 2 (6) | −15 (−20) Pleasant Not angry Reflective | −48 (−41) Deliberate Precise Orderly | 35 (29) Curious Inventive Quick wit |
| Harm avoidance | −54 (−65) Bold Not shy Cheerful | 71 (71) Fearful Worrying Gloomy | −8 (−19) Trusting | −9 (−15) Painstaking | −10 (−21) Broadly interested |
| Reward dependence | 36 (44) Sociable Warm Affectionate | 10 (−8) | 42 (46) Sympathetic Responsive Sensitive | 2 (5) | 25 (34) Open Sentimental Not shallow |
| Persistence | 20 (10) Active Spunky Energetic | −9 (2) | 7 (4) | 62 (31) Conscientious Achieving Not shifty | −4 (2) |

**Character**

| | | | | | |
|---|---|---|---|---|---|
| Self-directed | 27 (35)<br>Assertive<br>Forceful<br>Bossy | −69 (−75)<br>Vulnerable<br>Self-pity<br>Incompetent | 33 (43)<br>Accepting<br>Not blaming | 46 (29)<br>Responsible<br>Planful<br>Organized | 5 (16) |
| Cooperative | 21 (32)<br>Kind<br>Congenial | −21 (−38)<br>Touchy<br>Cynical<br>Hostile | 66 (64)<br>Helpful<br>Forgiving<br>Tender | 17 (33)<br>Dependable<br>Principled | 23 (25)<br>Tolerant<br>Thoughtful<br>Receptive |
| Self-transcendent | 26 (25)<br>Spontaneous<br>Natural<br>Humorous | 4 (−2) | 8 (7) | −3 (13) | 38 (12)<br>Imaginative<br>Artistic<br>Insightful |

*Note.* Correlations between the TCI and Costa and McCrae's NEO factors in a sample of college students (*N* = 803), followed by those in a sample of psychiatric patients (in parentheses; *N* = 136), are shown. Adjectives are based on analyses of discriminating descriptors of the five-factor model (John 1990) and joint factor analysis of the five- and seven-factor models (C. R. Cloninger et al. 1993, unpublished data).

**Table 3–10.**  Tridimensional Personality Questionnaire (TPQ) temperament profile of patients with different anxiety disorders compared with general-population control subjects

| Subject diagnosis | *n* | TPQ temperament dimensions | | |
| --- | --- | --- | --- | --- |
| | | Harm avoidance | Novelty seeking | Reward dependence[a] |
| Anxiety disorders | | | | |
| Generalized anxiety | 12 | 19.4* | 16.3 | 20.2 |
| Panic disorder | 18 | 20.3* | 15.4 | 21.3 |
| Panic with agoraphobia | 33 | 24.8* | 15.3 | 19.0 |
| Social phobia | 21 | 22.8* | 13.2 | 15.3* |
| Obsessional | 25 | 22.4* | 13.0 | 22.0* |
| | 32 | 20.8* | 15.3 | 18.8 |
| Control subjects | 1,019 | 12.0 | 13.0 | 18.9 |
| | | (SD = 5.9) | (SD = 5.0) | (SD = 4.0) |

*Note.*  TPQ values are means.
[a]Reward dependence in the publications from which the data in this table were derived comprised four scales, including persistence. In the study of 32 obsessional subjects, Summerfeldt and co-workers (1993) found RD134 = 13.2 and persistence RD2 = 5.6 (not different from those in control subjects); information in Pfohl's obsessive-compulsive disorder (OCD) study about the persistence subscale has been requested but is not yet available.
*P < .05.
*Source.*  Cowley et al. 1993 (generalized anxiety and panic disorder); Saviotti et al. 1991 (panic with agoraphobia); M. E. Tancer and R. N. Golden, abstract for Society of Biological Psychiatry, written communication, 1993 (social phobia); Pfohl et al. 1990 (25 OCD); L. J. Summerfeldt, M. Richter, and R. M. Bagby, written communication, November 1993 (32 OCD).

possibly persistence (Cloninger et al. 1994; Kleifield et al. 1993). Four independent studies have confirmed these predictions, as summarized in Table 3–11. All eating disorder patients are high in harm avoidance, but those with both anorexia and bulimia tend to be especially fearful (Bulik et al. 1992). Bulimic patients are also high in novelty seeking, whereas restrictive anorexic patients are also high in persistence. Discriminant analysis was used by Cynthia

**Table 3–11.** Tridimensional Personality Questionnaire (TPQ) temperament profiles of patients with subtypes of eating disorders

| Study | Eating disorder subtype | n | TPQ temperament dimensions | | | |
|---|---|---|---|---|---|---|
| | | | Harm avoidance | Novelty seeking | Reward dependence | Persistence |
| Kleifield et al. (1993) | Restrictive anorexia | 24 | 18.6* | 13.2 | 13.2 | 6.9* |
| | Anorexia + hx bulimia | 20 | 21.6* | 16.9* | 13.5 | 5.8 |
| | Bulimia + hx anorexia | 15 | 17.7* | 19.4* | 11.9 | 5.7 |
| | Bulimia | 22 | 20.5 | 18.5* | 13.3 | 5.3 |
| Brewerton et al. (1993) | Restrictive anorexia | 27 | 21.3* | 12.9 | 13.0 | 6.7* |
| | Bulimia + hx anorexia | 10 | 19.6* | 18.3* | 13.5 | 5.4 |
| | Bulimia | 110 | 20.0* | 18.1* | 14.3 | 6.1 |
| Waller et al. (1991) | Bulimia | 27 | 16.6* | 17.9* | 12.1* | 6.3 |
| Bulik et al. (1992) | Restrictive anorexia | 29 | 18.9* | 14.8 | 15.6* | 6.9* |
| | Anorexia + bulimia | 20 | 25.3* | 14.2 | 13.6 | 5.6 |
| | Bulimia | 32 | 21.2* | 17.7* | 14.0 | 5.9 |
| Control subjects | | 1,019 | 12.0 (SD = 5.9) | 13.0 (SD = 5.0) | 13.4 (SD = 3.4) | 5.5 (SD = 1.9) |

*Note.* TPQ values are means. hx = history of. Restrictive anorexic patients are consistently high in harm avoidance and persistence, and bulimic patients are consistently high in harm avoidance and novelty seeking.

Bulik and her associates in New Zealand to compare the classification accuracy of different psychometric batteries, including the
Eating Disorders Inventory, MMPI, Revised Symptom Checklist–
90 (SCL-90-R), and the TPQ (Table 3–12). The 12 TPQ subscales
were able to classify individuals by subtype of eating disorder about
as well as the Eating Disorders Inventory and better than the MMPI
and SCL-90-R.

## Starting and Stopping Cigarette Smoking

The initiation and cessation of cigarette smoking have been considered to be influenced by multiple processes. High novelty seeking, as an indicator of behavior activation, is predicted to be
a major determinant of the initiation of smoking, whereas high
harm avoidance is associated with difficulty terminating habits
maintained by positive reinforcement. Pomerleau and co-workers
(1992) found that smokers were higher in novelty seeking and

**Table 3–12.**  Accuracy of classification of four psychometric batteries
via discriminant analysis in women with eating disorders

| Battery | κ | Anorexia nervosa | Anorexia and bulimia | Bulimia nervosa |
|---|---|---|---|---|
| | | Correct classification (%) | | |
| EDI | | | | |
| Complete | .63 | 100 | 59 | 63 |
| No bulimia scale | .36 | 55 | 59 | 60 |
| TPQ | .58 | 81 | 67 | 72 |
| MMPI | .46 | 77 | 73 | 50 |
| SCL-90-R | .36 | 59 | 65 | 52 |

*Note.*  EDI = Eating Disorders Inventory; TPQ = Tridimensional Personality
Questionnaire; MMPI = Minnesota Multiphasic Personality Inventory;
SCL-90-R = Revised Symptom Checklist–90. The TPQ has highest discrim-
inant power of all batteries, including the EDI, when items pathognomonic
for bulimia are omitted.
*Source.*  Data derived from Bulik et al. 1992.

persistence than control subjects regardless of gender (Table 3–13). In addition, female smokers ranked higher in harm avoidance and male smokers ranked lower in reward dependence as a group. However, only high harm avoidance was associated with measures of nicotine dependence or addiction, indicating difficulty stopping (Table 3–14). These findings support the theoretical prediction that different processes are involved in the initiation, maintenance, and cessation of smoking and other motivated behaviors. Regular cigarette smokers combine characteristics that are dissociated in bulimic (i.e., novelty seeking) and restrictive anorexic (i.e., persistence) individuals.

# Personality Profiles Associated With Subtypes of Alcoholism

Some of the most extremely dysfunctional personality disorders are observed in individuals in treatment centers for the chemically

**Table 3–13.** Tridimensional Personality Questionnaire (TPQ) temperament profile of cigarette smokers without associated psychiatric disorder

| Subjects | n | TPQ temperament dimensions | | | |
|---|---|---|---|---|---|
| | | Harm avoidance | Novelty seeking | Reward dependence | Persistence |
| Women | | | | | |
| Smokers | 119 | 14.8* | 16.8* | 14.6 | 8.2* |
| Control subjects | 350 | 12.8 | 13.0 | 15.7 | 6.5 |
| Men | | | | | |
| Smokers | 121 | 11.5 | 17.2* | 11.5* | 7.7* |
| Control subjects | 326 | 10.5 | 13.7 | 14.1 | 6.5 |

*Note.* TPQ values are means.
*$P < .05$.
*Source.* Data derived from Pomerleau et al. 1992.

**Table 3–14.**  Relationship between Tridimensional Personality
Questionnaire (TPQ) scores and nicotine dependence
or difficulty stopping smoking

| Variable among smokers | n | Correlations (×100) with TPQ temperament dimensions | | | |
|---|---|---|---|---|---|
| | | Harm avoidance | Novelty seeking | Reward dependence | Persistence |
| Nicotine dependence[a] | | | | | |
| Women | 119 | 33* | −11 | 13 | 5 |
| Men | 121 | 4 | 3 | −3 | 7 |
| Addictive smoking[b] | | | | | |
| Women | 119 | 28* | −8 | 11 | 16 |
| Men | 121 | 43* | −1 | 0 | 0 |

[a]Nicotine dependence measured by Fagerstrom Tolerance Questionnaire.
[b]"Addictive" smoking measured by Russell Motives for Smoking Questionnaire, indicating difficulty stopping smoking.
*$P < .05$.
*Source.*   Data derived from Pomerleau et al. 1992.

dependent. This is illustrated by the profiles of patients hospitalized for chemical dependency in Oklahoma (Nixon and Parsons 1990). This treatment sample had extremely high scores and reduced variance on all temperament dimensions reported (Table 3–15); these patients are more than two standard deviations above the means for each temperament dimension for individuals in the general population (see Table 3–19 later in this chapter). Fortunately, such extreme variants are not characteristic of all individuals who abuse substances, but indicate that some treatment centers may overrepresent chronic cases with multiple temperament deviations because these combined deviations induce chronicity. Nevertheless, the findings in this extreme sample show that the TPQ measures variability across a wide range without much difficulty from ceiling effects.

Cannon and co-workers (1993) studied hospitalized male vet-

**Table 3–15.** Tridimensional Personality Questionnaire (TPQ) scores for inpatients ($N = 257$) recruited from chemical dependency treatment units in Oklahoma

| Gender | n | TPQ temperament dimensions | | |
|--------|---|--------------------|--------------------|-------------------------------|
| | | Harm avoidance | Novelty seeking | Reward dependence and persistence |
| Men | 169 | $25.4 \pm 3.1$ | $27.9 \pm 3.4$ | $27.0 \pm 3.1$ |
| Women | 88 | $26.5 \pm 3.8$ | $28.4 \pm 3.3^a$ | $27.7 \pm 3.1$ |

*Note.* TPQ values are means ± standard deviations. Note the extremely high scores and restricted variances on all dimensions in this treatment sample.
[a]Women rank higher than men in harm avoidance ($P < .05$).
*Source.* Data derived from Nixon and Parsons 1990.

erans with alcohol dependence and examined the relationships between personality and the features of type 2 alcoholism, which is associated with early onset of both polydrug abuse and antisocial behavior (Cloninger 1987a; Cloninger et al. 1981). Novelty seeking was positively correlated with antisocial behavior and early-onset type 2 alcohol abuse (Table 3–16). Likewise, in a study of 173 adult male drug users (Nagoshi et al. 1992), the validity of each considered dimension of the TPQ was also supported by studies with the EPQ, the Buss-Durkee Hostility-Guilt Inventory, the SCL-90, and other tests: novelty seeking was correlated with impulsivity, aggression, and criminality; harm avoidance was correlated with introversion, neuroticism, low venturesomeness, and high psychological distress; and reward dependence was correlated with extraversion, empathy, and low psychoticism.

Whereas individuals with type 2 alcoholism with early onset and antisocial behavior are associated with high novelty seeking and low harm avoidance in treatment (Cannon et al. 1993) and longitudinal studies (Cloninger et al. 1988), those with a history of prolonged abstinence are associated with high harm avoidance. Whipple and Noble (1991) observed increased harm avoidance in alcoholic fathers with a history of at least 2 years of sobriety compared with fathers with a negative personal and family history of

**Table 3–16.** Relationship between Tridimensional Personality
Questionnaire (TPQ) scores and antisocial behavior and
alcohol subtype in male veterans hospitalized for alcohol
dependence ($N$ = 303)

| Clinical variable[a] | Correlation ($\times$ 100) with TPQ temperament dimensions | | | |
|---|---|---|---|---|
| | Harm avoidance | Novelty seeking | Reward dependence | Persistence |
| Type 2 alcoholism | 15 | 38* | −10 | −15 |
| Childhood misconduct | 8 | 37* | −11 | −6 |
| Military misconduct | 10 | 35* | −16 | −6 |
| Criminal arrests | 13 | 18 | −9 | −3 |
| Polydrug use | 16 | 30* | −12 | −18 |
| Age at onset of alcoholism | −10 | −24* | −5 | 2 |

[a]Clinical variables coded as number of designated antisocial features, number
of drugs, and number of symptoms characteristic of type 2 alcoholism (onset
of alcohol abuse before age 26 years, including hospitalization, arrests or
fights, almost daily drunkenness after onset of first problem).
*$P$ < .001.
*Source.* Data derived from Cannon et al. 1993.

alcoholism (Table 3–17). Likewise, the sons also differed in harm
avoidance. These findings about novelty seeking and harm avoidance in the onset and abstinence of alcohol abuse correspond to
the findings about these same personality traits in the initiation
and cessation of smoking.

Alcoholic individuals with antisocial personality disorder are
expected to be associated with high novelty seeking, low harm
avoidance, and low reward dependence (Cloninger 1987b). A study
of family history of alcoholism in volunteers by Hesselbrock and
Hesselbrock (1992) confirmed the association of antisocial personality disorder, diagnosed according to DSM-III-R criteria (American Psychiatric Association 1987), with high novelty seeking and
possibly low harm avoidance (Table 3–18). However, this study also
revealed a strong effect of volunteer status on personality, an effect
that confounds many such studies in biological psychiatry. Before

**Table 3–17.** Tridimensional Personality Questionnaire (TPQ) (version 2) scores in sons of alcoholic fathers selected for Type 1 feature of at least 2 years of sobriety (A+) and sons of fathers with no personal or family history of alcoholism (A–) and in a survey of the general population in which the same version of the TPQ was used

| Subjects | n | TPQ temperament dimensions | | | |
| | | Harm avoidance | Novelty seeking | Reward dependence | Persistence |
|---|---|---|---|---|---|
| Fathers | | | | | |
| A+ | 18 | 10.2* | 16.2 | 11.3 | 8.8 |
| A– | 20 | 5.7 | 15.2 | 12.5 | 8.4 |
| | | | | | |
| Sons | | | | | |
| A+ | 18 | 13.9* | 17.1 | 11.4 | 8.1 |
| A– | 20 | 8.8 | 18.6 | 11.6 | 9.1 |
| | | | | | |
| General population | 1,236 | 12.4 (SD = 6.1) | 14.2 (SD = 14.2) | 11.7 (SD = 3.8) | 8.0 (SD = 2.7) |

*Note.* TPQ values are means. MANOVA and discriminant analysis revealed significant group differences in sons and fathers with both harm avoidance and novelty-seeking subscales.
*$P < .05$.
*Source.* Data for sons and fathers derived from Whipple and Noble 1991, and those for the general population survey derived from Waller et al. 1991.

the relationship between personality dimensions and personality disorders is examined, the importance of selection biases needs to be taken into account.

# Selection Bias From Recruitment Methods

The TPQ has been normed in a rigorous national area probability sampled in cooperation with the National Opinion Research Council (Cloninger et al. 1991). The means and standard deviations in this normative sample are representative of the general

**Table 3–18.** Relationship between Tridimensional Personality Questionnaire (TPQ) (version 2) temperament dimensions and personal diagnosis of antisocial personality disorder/family history of alcoholism in young men ($N = 91$) volunteering for research in response to advertisements and comparison with scores of general population control subjects

| Volunteer subgroup | $n$ | TPQ temperament dimensions | | | |
|---|---|---|---|---|---|
| | | **Harm avoidance** | **Novelty seeking** | **Reward dependence** | **Persistence** |
| ASP+/FH+ | 15 | 7.5 | 24.8[a] | 11.0 | 6.8 |
| ASP+/FH– | 19 | 8.6 | 26.2[a] | 11.2 | 7.9 |
| ASP–/FH+ | 29 | 10.7 | 20.4 | 12.3 | 7.9 |
| ASP–/FH– | 28 | 8.4 | 19.6 | 12.2 | 7.6 |
| Total volunteers | 91 | 9.0 | 22.1 | 11.8 | 7.6 |
| General population | 1,236 | 12.4 (SD = 6.1) | 14.2 (SD = 5.2) | 11.7 (SD = 3.8) | 8.0 (SD = 2.7) |

*Note.* TPQ values are means. ASP = antisocial personality disorder; FH = family history of alcoholism. This study used TPQ version 2, so control values are related to those for that version based on a survey of the general population (Waller et al. 1991). This version required a high school reading level and included items in the key of the persistence scale moved to other reward dependence scales in version 4, which has been distributed since 1987. Note that volunteers to advertisements for a study with quick payment of $100 as a group are more than one standard deviation higher in novelty seeking and half a standard deviation lower in harm avoidance than a sample representative of young men in the general population.
[a]ASP+ volunteers and ASP– volunteers differed significantly ($P < .05$).
*Source.* Data for 91 young men volunteering for research in response to advertisements derived from Hesselbrock and Hesselbrock 1992, and those for the general population derived from Waller et al. 1991.

noninstitutionalized adult population. Comparison of these general population values with those of control subjects ascertained by different selection methods permits evaluation of the role of personality in ascertainment processes. The scores in the general population and in various groups selected as normal control subjects in research studies are summarized in Table 3–19.

One major variable in selection is whether the subjects are identified as voluntary respondents to advertisements or are targeted members of a specific population (e.g., national area probability sample, membership in a registry, or consecutive admissions to a hospital unit). Accordingly, the first half of Table 3–19 reports scores for groups in which subjects were individually recruited from a specific target population; the second half of the table reports scores for groups in which subjects were self-selected volunteers responding to advertisements or optional requests. A second major variable is related to motivational inducements to participate, such as payment. A third variable is screening for personal and/or familial psychiatric disorder (healthy vs. any volunteer).

As can be seen in Table 3–19, population-based methods with minimal delayed payment and exclusion screening produce subjects with personality distributions comparable to those in the general population. However, offers of high payment to participate in demanding tasks or intoxication (e.g., Schuckit et al. 1990) produce a biased sample with high novelty seeking and low harm avoidance. Likewise, volunteers responding to advertisements about interesting experiences or optional requests are systematically higher in novelty seeking than the general population, whether or not they are paid. Furthermore, screening for mental health has the general effect of reducing harm avoidance scores substantially. Such selection biases can confound the interpretation of research in which personality is potentially a risk factor. Accordingly, the case-control design is problematic for studies of personality and its disorders.

## Population-Based Analyses of Personality Disorder

To avoid such selection biases, it is prudent to conduct studies of representative samples of a target population and then partition the whole population according to variables of interest. The relation-

**Table 3–19.** Mean Tridimensional Personality Questionnaire (TPQ) (version 4) scores in the general population and various groups selected as control subjects in research: population-based groups (i.e., individually recruited from target population) and self-selected (i.e., volunteer) groups

| Selection method | Study | Reference | n | TPQ temperament dimensions | | | |
|---|---|---|---|---|---|---|---|
| | | | | Harm avoidance | Novelty seeking | Reward dependence | Persistence |
| **Population-based** | | | | | | | |
| Minimal pay | National Area Probability Sample | Cloninger et al. (1991) | 1,019 | 12.0 (5.9) | 13.0 (5.0) | 13.4 (3.4) | 5.5 (1.9) |
| | National Area Probability Sample matched to young bulimic women by age/gender | Waller et al. (1991) | 128 women | 11.8 (5.6) | 14.5 (5.1) | 14.9 (3.4) | 6.2 (1.7) |
| | Medical-surgical hospital patients | Menza et al. (1990) | 20 | 11.6 (5.4) | 13.8 (4.2) | 19.5 (4.4) | |
| High pay | Healthy recruits for extensive battery of tests including intoxication | Schuckit et al. (1990) | 33 | 9.1 (5.2) | 17.4 (5.4) | 19.8 (4.7) | |

| | | | | | |
|---|---|---|---|---|---|
| **Self-selected** | | | | | |
| For pay | | | | | |
| Pfohl et al. (1990) | 35 | 10.3 (3.6) | 15.0 (3.6) | 19.1 (3.9) | |
| Zaninelli et al. (1992) | 25 | 8.3 (4.6) | 17.6 (4.1) | 20.7 (5.0) | |
| Cowley et al. (1993) | 21 | 10.2 (6.0) | 18.2 (3.8) | 20.0 (3.8) | |
| Tancer and Golden (1993) | 22 | 8.8 (3.6) | 16.2 (4.5) | 18.6 (3.8) | |
| Low pay | | | | | |
| Stallings et al. (in press) | 1,070 men | 10.5 (6.1) | 11.6 (4.8) | 12.2 (3.7) | 4.6 (2.1) |
| | 3,045 women | 12.9 (6.4) | 12.0 (4.8) | 13.2 (3.5) | 4.9 (2.1) |
| No pay | | | | | |
| Peterson et al. (1991) | 20 | 9.6 (5.3) | 19.0 (6.3) | 12.6 (3.0) | 4.2 (2.0) |
| Cloninger et al. (1994) | 803 | 14.0 (7.3) | 16.6 (5.6) | 14.7 (3.5) | 5.6 (2.1) |

Healthy volunteers to convenient advertisements for interesting experience and quick payment

Population-based volunteers to advertisement for twins older than 50 years of age (minimal and delayed pay)

Healthy volunteers as part of college psychology course (no payment)

Any volunteers as part of college psychology course (no payment)

ship between self-reported personality and personality disorder interviews in a consecutive series of psychiatric inpatients has recently been described (Svrakic et al. 1993). This study showed that the presence of any personality disorder was strongly determined by low scores in self-directedness and cooperativeness. Low reward dependence, high novelty seeking, or high harm avoidance predicted that the personality disorder, if present, was in DSM-III-R cluster A (odd), B (impulsive), or C (anxious), respectively. Each individual personality disorder category was defined as a function of the configuration of scores on all seven dimensions. In other words, traditional personality disorder variants can be defined in terms of a configural profile of genetically independent dimensions.

Similar results were obtained in a study of 23 affectively ill adolescents (Brent et al. 1990). In particular, adolescents in the impulsive cluster were much higher in novelty seeking than were other patients.

## Conclusions and Recommendations

The genetic architecture of personality has finally provided a definitive criterion for a rational taxonomy of personality. This etiologically based model is uniquely specified in terms of four dimensions of temperament (novelty seeking, harm avoidance, reward dependence, and persistence) and three dimensions of character (self-directedness, cooperativeness, self-transcendence). The convergent and discriminant validity of these measures is supported by a wide range of studies of normal and abnormal groups. Alternative measures of impulsiveness are composed of variable contributions from high novelty seeking, low harm avoidance, low persistence, and, rarely, low reward dependence. In contrast, alternative measures of compulsiveness are composed of variable contributions from high harm avoidance, low novelty seeking, high persistence, and, rarely, high reward dependence. Rather than a specialized test being developed for every situation, more systematic progress will result from inclusion of measurements based on the Tridimensional Personality Questionnaire and the Temperament and Character Inventory, because only these dimensions have been confirmed to be genetically homogeneous and independent. Additional measures should also be considered, but not to the exclusion of the TCI, which is a comprehensive and reliable index of the biogenetic structure of personality.

A comprehensive description and bibliography of the development and clinical use of the seven-factor model of temperament and character have been published elsewhere as a manual for the TCI that can be obtained from the author (Cloninger et al. 1994). The TCI manual also summarizes available data on the validity and psychometric properties of the TCI subscales, and on the neurocognitive and neurochemical correlates of each dimension, and provides illustrative case reports about assessment and clinical management. Now that a sound etiologically based model is available, future work on clinical assessment and management using the TCI should be fruitful.

# References

Adamec RE: Anxious personality in the cat: ontogeny and physiology, in Psychopathology and the Brain. Edited by Carroll BJ, Barrett JE. New York, Raven, 1991, pp 153–168

American Psychiatric Association: Diagnostic and Statistical Manual of Mental Disorders, 3rd Edition, Revised. Washington, DC, American Psychiatric Association, 1987

Bagby RM, Parker JDA, Joffe RT: Confirmatory factor analysis of the Tridimensional Personality Questionnaire. Personality and Individual Differences 13:1245–1246, 1992

Brent DA, Zelenak JP, Bukstein O, et al: Reliability and validity of the Structured Interview for Personality Disorders in adolescents. J Am Acad Child Adolesc Psychiatry 29:349–354, 1990

Brewerton TD, Hand LD, Bishop ER Jr: The Tridimensional Personality Questionnaire in eating disorder patients. International Journal of Eating Disorders 14:213–218, 1993

Brown SL, Svrakic DM, Przybeck TR, et al: The relationship of personality to mood and anxiety states: a dimensional approach. J Psychiatr Res 26:197–211, 1992

Bulik CM, Sullivan PF, Weltzin TE, et al: Temperament in eating disorders. Written manuscript of paper presented at the Royal Australia and New Zealand College of Psychiatrists, Christchurch, New Zealand, September 1992

Cannon DS, Clark LA, Leeka JK, et al: A reanalysis of the Tridimensional Personality Questionnaire (TPQ) and its relation to Cloninger's Type 2 alcoholism. Psychological Assessment 5:62–66, 1993

Carroll BJ, Barrett JE (eds): Psychopathology and the Brain. New York, Raven, 1991

Cloninger CR: A unified biosocial theory of personality and its role in the development of anxiety states. Psychiatric Developments 4:167–226, 1986

Cloninger CR: Neurogenetic adaptive mechanisms in alcoholism. Science 236:410–416, 1987a

Cloninger CR: A systematic method for clinical description and classification of personality variants. Arch Gen Psychiatry 44:573–588, 1987b

Cloninger CR: Reply to Marvin Zuckerman (reply to letter). Arch Gen Psychiatry 45:503–504, 1988

Cloninger CR: Brain networks underlying personality development, in Psychopathology and the Brain. Edited by Carroll BJ, Barrett JE. New York, Raven, 1991, pp 183–208

Cloninger CR, Bohman M, Sigvardsson S: Inheritance of alcohol abuse: cross-fostering analysis of adopted men. Arch Gen Psychiatry 38: 861–868, 1981

Cloninger CR, Martin RL, Guze SB, et al: Diagnosis and prognosis in schizophrenia. Arch Gen Psychiatry 40:15–25, 1985

Cloninger CR, Sigvardsson S, Bohman M: Childhood personality predicts alcohol abuse in young adults. Alcohol Clin Exp Res 12:494–505, 1988

Cloninger CR, Przybeck TR, Svrakic DM: The Tridimensional Personality Questionnaire: U.S. normative data. Psychol Rep 69:1047–1057, 1991

Cloninger CR, Svrakic DM, Przybeck TR: A psychobiological model of temperament and character. Arch Gen Psychiatry 50:975–990, 1993

Cloninger CR, Przybeck TR, Svrakic DM, et al: The Temperament and Character Inventory (TCI): A Guide to Its Development and Use. St Louis, MO, Washington University Center for the Psychobiology of Personality, 1994

Costa PT Jr, McCrae RR: Trait psychology comes of age. Nebr Symp Motiv 39:169–204, 1991

Cowley DS, Roy-Byrne PP, Greenblatt DJ, et al: Personality and benzodiazepine sensitivity in anxious patients and control subjects. Psychiatry Res 47:151–162, 1993

Digman JM: Five robust trait dimensions: development, stability, and utility. J Pers 57:195–214, 1989

Earleywine M, Finn PR, Peterson JB, et al: Factor structure and correlates of the Tridimensional Personality Questionnaire. J Stud Alcohol 53:233–238, 1992

Eaves L, Eysenck HJ: The nature of extraversion: a genetical analysis. J Pers Soc Psychol 32:102–112, 1975

Eysenck HJ, Eysenck SBG: Manual of the Eysenck Personality Questionnaire. London, Hodder & Stoughton, 1976

Gough HG: Manual for the California Personality Inventory. Palo Alto, CA, Consulting Psychologists Press, 1969

Gray JA: A critique of Eysenck's theory of personality, in A Model for Personality. Edited by Eysenck HJ. New York, Springer-Verlag, 1981, pp 246–276

Heath AC, Martin NG: Psychoticism as a dimension of personality: a multivariate genetic test of Eysenck and Eysenck's psychoticism construct. J Pers Soc Psychol 58:1–11, 1990

Heath AC, Cloninger CR, Martin NG: Testing a model for the genetic structure of personality: a comparison of the personality systems of Cloninger and Eysenck. J Pers Soc Psychol 66:762–775, 1994

Hesselbrock MN, Hesselbrock VM: Relationship of family history, antisocial personality disorder and personality traits in young men at risk for alcoholism. J Stud Alcohol 53:619–625, 1992

Joffe RT, Bagby RM, Levitt AJ, et al: The Tridimensional Personality Questionnaire in major depression. Am J Psychiatry 150:959–960, 1993

John OP: The search for basic dimensions of personality: review and critique. Advances in Psychological Assessment 7:1–37, 1990

Kendell R: The choice of diagnostic criteria for biological research. Arch Gen Psychiatry 39:1334–1339, 1982

Kleifield EI, Sunday S, Hurt S, et al: The tridimensional personality theory: application to subgroups of eating disorders. Compr Psychiatry 34:249–253, 1993

Kozeny J, Kubicka L, Prochazkova Z: Psychometric properties of the Czech version of Cloninger's Tridimensional Personality Questionnaire. Personality and Individual Differences 10:1253–1259, 1989

MacAndrews C: The differentiation of male alcoholic outpatients from nonalcoholic psychiatric outpatients by means of the MMPI. Quarterly Journal of Studies on Alcohol 26:238–246, 1965

McCourt WF, Gurrera RJ, Cutter HS: Sensation seeking and novelty seeking. Are they the same? J Nerv Ment Dis 181:309–312, 1993

Menza MA, Forman NE, Goldstein HS, et al: Parkinson's disease, personality, and dopamine. J Neuropsychiatry Clin Neurosci 2:282–287, 1990

Nagoshi CT, Walter D, Muntaner C, et al: Validation of the Tridimensional Personality Questionnaire in a sample of male drug users. Personality and Individual Differences 13:401–409, 1992

Nixon SJ, Parsons OA: Cloninger's tridimensional theory of personality: construct validity in a sample of college students. Personality and Individual Differences 10:1261–1267, 1989

Nixon SJ, Parsons OA: Application of the Tridimensional Personality Questionnaire to a population of alcoholics and other substance abusers. Alcohol Clin Exp Res 14:513–517, 1990

Perna G, Bernardeschi L, Caldirola D, et al: Personality dimension in panic disorder: state versus traits issues. New Trends in Experimental and Clinical Psychiatry 8:49–54, 1992

Peterson JB, Weiner D, Pihl RO, et al: The Tridimensional Personality Questionnaire and the inherited risk for alcoholism. Addict Behav 16:549–554, 1991

Pfohl B, Black D, Noyes R Jr, et al: A test of the tridimensional personality theory: association with diagnosis and platelet imipramine binding in obsessive-compulsive disorder. Biol Psychiatry 28:41–46, 1990

Pomerleau CS, Pomerleau OF, Flessland KA, et al: Relationship of Tridimensional Personality Questionnaire scores and smoking variables in female and male smokers. J Subst Abuse 4:143–154, 1992

Saviotti FM, Grandi S, Savron G, et al: Characterological traits of recovered patients with panic disorder and agoraphobia. J Affect Disord 23:113–117, 1991

Schalling D, Edman G: Personality and Vulnerability to Psychopathology: The Development of the Karolinska Scales of Personality (KSP). Stockholm, Karolinska Hospital, 1986

Schalling D, Cronholm B, Åsberg M, et al: Ratings of psychic and somatic anxiety indicants—interrater reliability and relations to personality variables. Acta Psychiatr Scand 49:353–368, 1973

Schuckit MA, Irwin M, Mahler HI: Tridimensional Personality Questionnaire scores of sons of alcoholic and nonalcoholic fathers. Am J Psychiatry 147:481–487, 1990

Selzer ML: The Michigan Alcoholism Screening Test: a quest for a new diagnostic instrument. Am J Psychiatry 127:1653–1658, 1971

Sjobring H: Personality structure and development: a model and its application. Acta Psychiatr Scand Suppl 244:1–204, 1973

Stallings MC, Hewitt JK, Cloninger CR, et al: Factor structure of the Tridimensional Personality Questionnaire: three or four primary personality dimensions? J Pers Soc Psychol (in press)

Strakowski SM, Stoll AL, Tohen M, et al: The Tridimensional Personality Questionnaire as a predictor of six-month outcome in first-episode mania. Psychiatry Res 48:1–8, 1993

Strandbygaard N, Jensen HH: Cloninger's biosocial personality theory. Nordisk Psykiatrisk Tidsskrift 46:345–350, 1992

Svrakic DM, Przybeck TR, Cloninger CR: Further contribution to the conceptual validity of the unified biosocial model of personality: U.S. and Yugoslav data. Compr Psychiatry 32:195–209, 1991

Svrakic DM, Przybeck TR, Cloninger CR: Mood states and personality traits. J Affect Disord 24:217–226, 1992

Svrakic DM, Whitehead C, Przybeck TR, et al: Differential diagnosis of personality disorders by the seven-factor model of temperament and character. Arch Gen Psychiatry 50:991–999, 1993

Takeuchi M, Yoshino A, Kato M, et al: Reliability and validity of the Japanese version of the Tridimensional Personality Questionnaire among university students. Compr Psychiatry 34:273–279, 1993

Waller NG, Zavala JD: Evaluating the Big Five. Psychological Inquiry 4:131–135, 1993

Waller NG, Lilienfeld SO, Tellegen A, et al: The Tridimensional Personality Questionnaire: structural validity and comparison with the Multidimensional Personality Questionnaire. Multivariate Behavioral Research 26:1–23, 1991

Wetzel RD, Knesevich MA, Brown SL, et al: Correlates of Tridimensional Personality Questionnaire scales with selected Minnesota Multiphasic Personality Inventory scales. Psychol Rep 71:1027–1038, 1992

Whipple SC, Noble EP: Personality characteristics of alcoholic fathers and their sons. J Stud Alcohol 52:331–337, 1991

Zaninelli RM, Porjesz B, Begleiter H: The Tridimensional Personality Questionnaire in males at high and low risk for alcoholism. Alcohol Clin Exp Res 16:68–70, 1992

Zuckerman M: Sensation seeking: a comparative approach to a human trait. Behav Brain Sci 7:413–471, 1984

Zuckerman M, Kuhlman DM, Joireman J, et al: A comparison of three structural models of pesonality: the Big Three, the Big Five, and the Alternative Five. J Pers Soc Psychol 65:757–768, 1993

# 4

# Cognitive Science Models of Compulsivity and Impulsivity

## Dan J. Stein, M.B.

ognitive science is a multidisciplinary arena that has re-placed behaviorism as the predominant paradigm in the psychological sciences (H. Gardner 1985). Central to the field are computational models of the mind, but its concepts and methodologies are drawn from cognitive psychology, artificial intelligence, linguistics, neuroscience, anthropology, and philosophy (Posner 1990). In recent years, an intersection between cognitive and clinical science has been more fully articulated (Stein 1994; Stein and Young 1992). This intersection has itself been an integrative one, with both psychoanalytically (Horowitz 1991; Peterfreund 1971) and cognitive-behaviorally (Beck 1967; Ellis 1962) oriented clinicians having applied cognitivist constructs to a variety of clinical phenomena (Stein 1992a, 1992b).

In this chapter I sketch a cognitive science approach to the clinical phenomena of compulsivity and impulsivity. To do this, I begin by considering cognitive science models in general.

# Cognitive Science Architectures

The models that cognitive scientists use may be divided into two broad categories: those with *symbolic* architectures and those with *connectionist* architectures. The elements of symbolic systems are symbols, which are stored in associative structures. The most widely employed of these structures is the *schema*. Schema theory posits that schemas are organizations of conceptually related elements representing a prototypic abstraction of a complex concept; it is further posited that schemas gradually develop from past experience and guide the organization of new information (Thorndyke and Hayes-Roth 1979). The elements of connectionist systems, on the other hand, are simplified and schematized neurons that are interconnected in a network. Response of the network again depends both on current input and on past learning. A variety of these parallel processing models have been developed (Rumelhart et al. 1986).

Although there are those who insist that only one or the other of these paradigms is accurate, the two kinds of models can also be seen as complementary. Schema architectures allow a top-down approach to the mind, whereas connectionist models are more suited to a bottom-up approach. Neural networks can be conceptualized as providing a detailed, neurobiologically consistent formalization of many of the properties of schemas. In this chapter, however, I focus on schema models, because there has been less work on neural network models of compulsivity and impulsivity.

In the schema-based view, it is possible to dissect out cognitive structures, cognitive processes, and cognitive events (Ingram and Kendall 1986). For example, a particular cognitive module (structure) may be responsible for generating verbs, it may be activated (process), and this may result in the articulation of a specific word (event). This kind of analysis is useful in generating information-processing models of several kinds of cognitive activity.

Schema-based architectures can also be used to understand psychopathology and psychotherapy. For example, in depression, there may be a negative self-schema (structure) that is triggered by loss (process), resulting in pessimistic statements and feelings (events). In psychotherapy, the depressed patient is encouraged to develop and use alternative schemas. Although schemas are a "cognitive" construct, the application of schema theory to clinical phenomena necessarily results in the incorporation of affect into these clinical cognitive science models. Such models have been employed to analyze a variety of clinical disorders, including compulsive and impulsive disorders (Ingram and Kendall 1986; Stein and Young 1992).

# Compulsivity

## Cognitive Structures

In obsessive-compulsive disorder (OCD), the psychological events of interest within a cognitive science framework are obsessive thoughts and compulsive actions. The phenomenology of these events is discussed in more detail in Chapter 1 in this volume. The focus in this discussion is on the symptoms of OCD rather than the compulsive symptoms seen in obsessive-compulsive personality disorder or other compulsive conditions, because these may be mediated by different cognitive structures and processes. An immediate question is the nature of the underlying cognitive structures that are in fact instrumental in producing the events of OCD.

One of the first to tackle this question was, of course, Freud. He suggested that "obsessional neurosis" (his term for what is now referred to as OCD) was characterized by regression to a pregenital psychic organization, in which there were excessive anal impulses and a harsh superego (Freud 1913/1958; Freud 1926/1959). In more cognitive terms, when particular structures are activated, the production of OCD symptoms follows. However, Freud's model of OCD is not always easily reformulated in cognitivist terms. Whereas cognitive models emphasize psychological structures, Freud's model of psychic structures is based on a metapsychology that emphasizes psychic energetics. Regression does not simply entail activation of early psychological structures; rather, it also implies a particular balance of mental forces. Cognitive science makes no such attempt to reduce cognitive models to the laws of physics.

Freud suggested that the particular psychic organization that characterizes obsessional neurosis may have an important constitutional component (Freud 1913/1958). From the viewpoint of cognitive science, it is similarly possible to turn to neurobiology to provide information about the specific features of the cognitive structures that mediate OCD symptoms.

Neurobiology has in fact provided several bottom-up guidelines. The concept of fixed action patterns in neuroethology, for example, appears directly applicable to OCD. Fixed action patterns are specific motor sequences, such as grooming behaviors, that are present in all members of a species. These patterns are highly conserved and are mediated by lower brain centers. They are triggered by environmental events (e.g., exposure to dirt leads to increased grooming). At times, behaviors governed by fixed action patterns may be considered pathological. For example, in the presence of conflicting environmental stimuli, a repetitive partial motor sequence may emerge. Alternatively, genetic factors may result in an overly low threshold for the emergence of a fixed action pattern. Thus, for example, dogs with acral lick dermatitis lick their extremities excessively, even in the absence of increased exposure to dirt (Rapoport et al. 1992; Stein et al. 1992).

There is some evidence that it is useful to conceptualize OCD in terms of similar biologically based structures. The symptoms of OCD are not only relatively universal but also relatively specific, suggesting that genetically determined behavioral sequences may be relevant to the disorder. Furthermore, many symptoms are reminiscent of repetitive grooming behaviors (e.g., hand washing). Other symptoms may be more related to nesting (e.g., hoarding) or guarding (e.g., checking) behaviors.

The neurobiology of these repetitive behaviors in animals and in humans converges, providing the strongest support for this hypothesis. Serotonin has been found to play an important role in mediating grooming behaviors in animals, acral lick dermatitis in dogs, and OCD symptoms in humans (Rapoport et al. 1992; Stein et al. 1992). In addition, the basal ganglia may have a central role in both grooming behaviors and OCD symptoms.

## Cognitive Processes

Ordinarily, the structures that mediate repetitive grooming behaviors are not activated in humans. The question arises, then, of the nature of the cognitive processes that mediate their activation in patients with OCD.

Under normal conditions, ruminative thoughts are in fact experienced fairly often (Martin and Tesser 1989). One trigger appears to be goal frustration, which leads to repetitive attempts to produce goal completion. This cybernetic process of determining the difference between current state and goal state and then providing feedback that enables adjustment of original plans is clearly central in day-to-day executive function.

If sufficiently intrusive and intense, ruminations may be pathological. A trigger for such thoughts may be severe frustration (e.g., loss of a loved one, with resultant obsessive thoughts about that person). It is important to note that ruminations may involve both automatic and controlled processes (Martin and Tesser 1989). Thus, a person who has lost a close relative may try to analyze the implications of this loss and to form new strategies and plans. At the same time, however, this person may be subject to unpredictable and dysphoric images of the lost relative. These intrusive events continue until new schemas of the relationship between the self and the lost other are formed (Horowitz 1989).

Neuropsychiatric research on OCD is consistent with the presence of impairments that may be related to pathological rumination. Several neuropsychological studies have shown, for example, that compared with psychiatrically healthy control subjects, OCD patients have increased difficulty on tests of cognitive set–shifting (e.g., Wisconsin Card Sorting Test, verbal fluency) (Head et al. 1989; Stein et al. 1994). Similarly, electrophysiological findings in OCD are consistent with overaroused and overfocused attention (Towey et al. 1990). Also, ruminations may be exacerbated by the anchoring effect of anxiety—that is, increased anxiety in OCD may reinforce rumination.

Neurotransmitter research provides important hints as to the biochemical basis of the cognitive processes that mediate ruminative processes. The serotonergic system has been hypothesized to signal the presence of possible harm (Depue and Spoont 1987), and it is possible to speculate that alterations in this system result in a change in the readiness with which an assessment of goal completion is made. OCD symptoms, for example, may begin after pregnancy (Neziroglu et al. 1992). It is possible that hormonal changes during pregnancy result in serotonergic dysfunction (Stein et al. 1993d). As a result there are increased attempts to get things "just right" and concomitant repetitive behaviors. The role of the serotonergic system in OCD is discussed more fully elsewhere in this volume (see Chapter 6). It is also possible that certain neuroanatomic factors lead to difficulties in determining whether goal completion has taken place. It may be hypothesized, for example, that orbitofrontal–basal ganglia feedback circuits are involved in determining the difference between current state and goal state and in adjusting initial plans (Stein and Hollander 1992). Dysfunction of these pathways might then be associated with an inability to determine whether goal completion has in fact occurred and consequent rumination. There is good evidence that these circuits are important in OCD, with a number of studies documenting hyperfrontality in OCD patients (Insel 1992).

In summary, distorted cognitive processes (with overestimation of harm) or deficient cognitive processes (with inability to determine goal completion) in OCD may mediate the repetitive activation of underlying behavioral patterns. Processing of internal representations in OCD often appears to overly emphasize internal cues. Although similar processes governing rumination are sometimes seen in response to certain environmental stimuli, in OCD such processes, and their associated structures, appear to have a strong link to specific neurobiological factors. Patients with OCD may readily articulate the content of certain schema propositions (e.g., explaining that there is danger they must get rid of). However, several processes may also take place outside of patients' awareness.

Finally, a number of other cognitive phenomena will typically be noted in OCD (and may even predispose to its development). These include attentional cuing (i.e., exaggerated focus on stimuli such as dirt), anchoring effects (i.e., increased rumination as a result of associated affect such as anxiety), and self-preoccupation (e.g., overresponsibility for actions).

# Impulsivity

## Cognitive Structures

The cognitive events associated with impulsivity include several clinical symptoms, such as impulsive aggression. These symptoms are discussed more fully in Chapter 1. Here, I address impulsive aggression as a unitary phenomenon, although to conceive of it as such is clearly an oversimplification (e.g., the discussion does not apply when impulsive aggression is secondary to another underlying psychiatric disorder). Once more, from a cognitive science perspective, an immediate question is the nature of the structures responsible for these phenomena.

Again, it is possible to turn to psychoanalysis for early attempts to answer this question. In the case of impulsive aggressive symptoms, the classical Freudian view emphasizes the importance of unconscious instincts with sexual and aggressive aims. Ordinarily, the ego attempts to control these instincts, but their associated psychic energy may manifest in a variety of everyday and pathological ways.

It may be argued that in his later work, Freud increasingly used cognitivist constructs, viewing anxiety, for example, as a signal (Stein 1992a). Certainly, later psychoanalysts have often employed overtly cognitivist theory. G. S. Klein (1954), for example, introduced the term "cognitive style" and contrasted obsessive and hysteric patients in terms of their general regulatory or control structures (R. W. Gardner et al. 1959).

In the cognitive-behavioral tradition, several authors have

similarly attempted to describe the structures that mediate impulsive aggressive behaviors in cognitivist terms (Ferguson and Rule 1983; Forgas 1986; Huesman 1988; Kendall and Braswell 1993; Lakoff 1987; Novaco and Welsh 1989). Application of schema theory to impulsive aggressive behaviors leads to the idea of a schema that governs the interpretation of certain environmental events in terms of anger and aggression and that suggests corresponding angry and aggressive behaviors as an optimal response.

Cognitivist authors have, for example, described "scripts" that govern aggressive behavior, in much the same way as cognitive psychologists have detailed scripts that govern, say, behavior in a restaurant. Like schemas, scripts order the interpretation of new events, making them quickly predictable and comprehensible. However, they also may lead to errors in information processing. Individual differences in aggressive behavior may be determined by variation in 1) the interpretation of environmental cues, 2) the contents of memory for aggressive scripts, and 3) the assessment of the aggressive script as appropriate and effective (Huesman 1988).

The question of whether aggressive schemas or scripts have a neurobiological basis is a controversial one. The idea of inherited neural patterns that mediate aggression has been accepted since Darwin. Furthermore, contemporary neuroscientists are able to provide information about the specific neurotransmitter systems and neuroanatomic structures that underpin these patterns. For example, laboratory research with animal models and clinical findings in patients with neurological disorders indicate that brain structures such as the limbic system and the hypothalamus mediate aggression (Bear 1991; Stein et al. 1995).

Nevertheless, it is unclear whether it is permissible to extrapolate findings from animal research and clinical findings in patients with gross neurological lesions to impulsivity. Subcortical structures that mediate programmed rage sequences are ordinarily under cortical control. Typical impulsive aggressive behaviors may differ substantially from behaviors that emerge after brain lesions. This caveat implies that we need also to focus on the cognitive processes that control aggressive behavior.

## Cognitive Processes

Under ordinary circumstances, structures that mediate impulsive aggression are triggered by a variety of factors. A particularly important factor may be the perception of threat to the self. An ordinarily nonviolent person may, for example, react with impulsive aggression during a mugging. Such impulsive aggression may also reach pathological proportions. In situations of chronic and severe threat (e.g., during times of economic hardship), there is likely to be a higher incidence of impulsive aggressive acts.

Alternatively, structures that mediate impulsive aggressive acts may be triggered excessively as a result of distortions or deficiencies in cognitive processes. In the absence of, for example, processes that adequately evaluate the outcome of aggressive scripts, such scripts are more likely to be triggered. Such evaluation would include 1) prediction of consequences of using the script, 2) assessment of whether the person is capable of executing the script, and 3) consideration of whether the script is congruent with internal standards (Hains and Ryan 1983; Huesman 1988). (See Gorenstein 1991 and Newman and Wallace 1993 for reviews of related literature on cognitive processes in psychopathic persons.)

Neuropsychiatric studies provide some evidence for dysfunction in cognitive processes in patients with increased impulsive aggression (Gorenstein 1991; Stein et al. 1995). A number of studies suggest that frontal lobe impairment plays a role in impulsivity, although many of these studies have been criticized for their methodological faults (see Kandel and Freed 1989 for review). We found that patients with increased histories of aggression had increased right-sided neurological soft signs, a pattern consistent with neuropsychological research linking left-hemisphere dysfunction with increased aggression (Stein et al. 1993b). Electrophysiological studies demonstrate impairment in timing-and-rhythm performance in impulsive subjects (Barratt 1987).

Neurotransmitter research again provides important clues about the biological basis for control of impulsive aggression. As mentioned earlier, the serotonin neurotransmitter system has been conceptualized as mediating harm-avoidant behaviors. Interestingly, there is strong evidence for the association of serotonin hypofunction and increased impulsive aggression (Stein et al. 1993c). The inborn setting of the cybernetic system determining impulsive responses is likely to vary from individual to individual (Kagan 1981). Although the genes responsible for this setting have not yet been elucidated, promising work is being done in this area (Brunner et al. 1993). Neurotransmitters other than serotonin may also be important (see Chapter 5). In addition, such factors as substance abuse will affect cognitive processes. One possiblity, for example, is that alcohol exerts significant effects on impulsive aggression via the serotonergic system.

In summary, distorted cognitive processes (with underestimation of harm) or deficient cognitive processes (with inability to evaluate outcome of aggressive scripts adequately) in impulsivity may mediate the activation of structures that govern aggressive behaviors. Processing of internal representations in impulsive aggression often appears to overly emphasize immediate external cues. Although the processes that govern the activation of aggressive scripts may have important neurobiological components, it is unlikely that these scripts are themselves fully biologically determined. Patients with impulsive aggression may readily articulate the content of certain schema propositions (e.g., explaining that it is important to respond to threat by attacking). However, several processes may also take place outside of patients' awareness. Finally, a number of other cognitive phenomena will typically be noted in impulsive aggression (and may even predispose to its development). These include attentional cuing (i.e., exaggerated focus on stimuli such as threat), anchoring effects (i.e., increased aggression as a result of associated affect such as anger), and self-preoccupation (e.g., lack of empathy for the other).

# Clinical Implications

As discussed earlier, cognitive science offers clinicians the advantages of an integrative multidisciplinary approach. This argument may be exemplified by considering the clinical implications of cognitive models of compulsivity and impulsivity. Although based on a cognitivist framework, these models allow for the incorporation of a range of modalities of assessment and treatment. A clinical vignette is provided to introduce and illustrate each section of the following discussion.

## Compulsivity

Andrew is an 18-year-old man who presented with symptoms of excessive hand washing, with consequent excoriation of his hands and fingers. This behavior had begun only recently, although Andrew recalled that as a child he had spent several hours each day lining up objects in his room in order to arrange them "just so." He explained that although he knew that he washed his hands too much and that this behavior was clearly interfering with his college work, the behavior was necessary in order to rid his mind of thoughts about becoming infected by dangerous germs.

As part of the clinical assessment, Andrew's psychiatrist asked in detail about Andrew's belief in germs: How did one come into contact with germs? How did contact result in infection? What were the consequences of infection? Andrew's answers indicated that in his thoughts about infection, he consistently overestimated the possibility of harm in day-to-day life. As part of the clinical examination, the psychiatrist completed a brief neurological soft score rating, which demonstrated that Andrew had a number of subtle deficits.

Andrew's psychiatrist suggested that clomipramine, a serotonergic antidepressant, would be helpful. At the same time, he encouraged Andrew to consider more carefully his thoughts about the harmfulness of germs. Andrew was "assigned" a homework project to discover more about such microorganisms. In addition, the psychiatrist encouraged Andrew to expose himself to the very stimuli that he feared most. For example, during their session, the psychiatrist touched his undersole and then playfully encouraged Andrew to shake his hand.

A cognitive science model of OCD suggests that, in addition to the diagnosis of symptoms, several other assessments may be useful. For example, patients should be assessed for cognitive distortions in their assessments of harm. Exaggeration of possible harm may be a suitable focus for psychotherapy. Patients should also be assessed for cognitive deficits. Neurological soft sign examination of OCD patients can be performed quickly and with good reliability (Hollander et al. 1990). Higher soft sign scores correlate with increased ventricular brain ratios (Stein et al. 1993a) and with decreased response to serotonin reuptake inhibitors (Hollander et al. 1991).

A cognitive science model of OCD implies that several forms of clinical intervention may be effective in this disorder. For example, pharmacotherapy may be used to change the setting of the cybernetic system with regard to the relevance of considerations of possible danger. Pharmacotherapy may also be useful in changing underlying mood processes that enhance compulsivity. Indeed, serotonin reuptake inhibitors are an important treatment modality in OCD (Zohar and Insel 1987).

Alternatively, cognitive-behavioral interventions can be used to alter the processes that trigger the cognitive structures responsible for OCD symptoms. Several studies have found that stimulus exposure with response prevention, for example, is likely to lead to a reduction in the ease with which OCD processes are activated (Baer and Minichiello 1990). Psychotherapy that employs metastatements about processes of harm exaggeration may also be useful (Salkovskis and Warwick 1988). The efficacy of such metastatements may be due to disruption of the automaticity of cognitive processes that mediate OCD symptoms.

## Impulsivity

Barry is a 26-year-old who agreed to see a psychiatrist after badly bruising his girlfriend, Beryl, in a fistfight. Barry admitted that this was not the first occasion on which this had happened; he noted that at times he was prone to explode with rage and that this was often followed by physical violence. In fact, a family practitioner had once referred Barry to a neurologist to make sure that he was not suffering from seizures, but a thorough workup had revealed no obvious pathology. Beryl had stayed with Barry partly because he inevitably felt extreme remorse shortly after his explosions, and at these times he would give her extra love and attention.

During the assessment, Barry's psychiatrist asked him to role-play situations that would lead him to lose his temper. It became clear that comments which Barry perceived as belittling his manhood would cause him anger. Barry viewed a wide range of comments in this light; for example, he might interpret a request from Beryl for help as a criticism that he was not there for her. As his anger escalated, Barry would feel that he had no options—the only possibility was to show "who was wearing the pants" by using force. A detailed history revealed that this behavior was particularly likely to occur during one of Barry's frequent bouts of depressed mood.

Barry's psychiatrist suggested that he begin fluoxetine in an attempt to control his depressed mood and impulsive aggressive behavior. At the same time, Barry was encouraged to monitor his feelings, to identify situations that increased his anger, and to consider alternative ways of defusing emotion and of solving conflicts. Continued practice in role playing allowed him to develop new patterns of thinking and behaving, which could then be used in his relationship with Beryl. Barry's psychiatrist emphasized that to "wear the pants" in the relationship with Beryl, Barry needed to develop the manly skills of close listening and careful problem solving.

A cognitive clinical approach to the assessment of impulsivity would again focus on the structures and processes that mediate symptomatic behaviors. For example, several role-play procedures have been developed that allow observation of aggressive cognitive scripts (Meichenbaum and Butler 1980; Novaco 1975). Manipulation of such procedures may yield information about selective encoding and retrieval of information in patients (Nasby and Kihlstrom 1986). Patients' responses to these procedures can be used as the basis for cognitive restructuring. Deficits in the ability to generate alternative strategies, to plan actions to meet a goal, and to anticipate consequences can also be assessed with specific psychometric tests (Novaco and Welsh 1989).

Once again, conceptualizing impulsivity in the context of a cognitive science model results in an eclectic approach to treatment. Pharmacotherapy may be useful in altering the threshold for threat perception and subsequent action (Stein et al. 1993c). Pharmacotherapy may also be important in changing underlying mood or thought dysfunction that enhances the activation of structures for aggression.

Alternatively, cognitive-behavioral interventions can be used to change the aggression threshold. Self-control techniques, for example, may reduce triggering of aggressive structures. Social skills training, including conflict-management techniques and problem-solving approaches, may be useful (Goldstein et al. 1979; Kendall and Braswell 1993). Meta-statements that analyze the sequence from cognitive interpretation to dysphoric affect to impulsive aggressive action may also be helpful (Linehan 1993). Although prognosis must remain guarded in patients with severe cognitive deficiencies, psychotherapy may reduce the automaticity of the processes underlying impulsive aggressive symptoms.

## Theoretical Implications

A central question raised by this volume is the definition of compulsivity and impulsivity. Neither of these concepts is, however, a unitary one. Compulsivity may be taken to refer to the symptoms of OCD, to various personality traits, or to underlying defense mechanisms. Similarly, it cannot be assumed that symptoms of impulsivity are always associated with impulsivity as defined by personality trait questionnaires, with impulsivity in role-play assessments, or with impulsivity on psychophysiological measures.

A cognitive science perspective may help shed light on the definitions of compulsivity and impulsivity by emphasizing the distinction between underlying structures, processes, and events.

For example, to clarify the concept of impulsivity, it is helpful to differentiate schemas with aggressive content, processes that inhibit or facilitate these schemas, and events that are aggressive or impulsive. Research on underlying structures and processes may help elucidate the nature of impulsivity even when the events that constitute clinical impulsivity are absent. Conversely, clinical impulsivity may result from the interplay of a range of different structures and processes.

The second central question raised by this volume is that of the relationship between compulsivity and impulsivity. Several kinds of answers have been proposed (Stein and Hollander 1993). The two constructs may be seen as diametrically opposed, or, alternatively, they may be viewed as similar, in that each implies a dysfunction of impulse control.

From a phenomenological perspective, compulsivity and impulsivity can be considered polar opposites insofar as the first is characterized by ruminative and stereotyped behavior to avoid harm, and the second is characterized by unconsidered and volatile behavior that may result in harm. Nevertheless, to the extent that both kinds of behaviors are repetitive but anxiety- or tension-reducing, with both ego-syntonic and ego-dystonic elements, there are perhaps some overlaps between compulsivity and impulsivity. A biological perspective might suggest that, in view of the serotonin hypofunction and hypofrontality associated with compulsivity and the serotonin hyperresponsivity and hyperfrontality associated with impulsivity, the two constructs are diametrically opposed (Hollander et al. 1993). Nevertheless, the complexity of the serotonergic system, and the possibility that changes in frontal lobe function are compensatory phenomena (Insel 1992), make this contrast more of a heuristic device than a definitive conclusion.

Psychodynamic authors have tended to view compulsivity and impulsivity as polar opposites. Since Freud, obsessional illness and hysteria have been theorized primarily in terms of their contrasts. Nevertheless, both obsessional illness and hysteria have been understood in terms of a model of psychic energy, and their similarity lies in the distorted expression of instincts. Only the form of repression differs in obsessional illness and hysteria: "The distinction between what occurs in hysteria and in an obsessional neurosis lies in the psychological processes which we can reconstruct behind the phenomena; the *result* is almost always the same, for the colourless mnemic content is rarely reproduced and plays no part in the patient's mental activity" (Freud 1909/1955, p. 196).

Certain cognitivist authors have similarly drawn sharp contrasts between compulsivity and impulsivity (Messer 1976; Messer and Schacht 1986; Miller 1989). In this chapter, however, the heterogeneity of both compulsivity and impulsivity have been emphasized. This heterogeneity may itself result in certain overlaps between the two categories. Some patients in both categories may be characterized by, for example, distorted cognitive processes relevant to harm assessment. Similarly, the behavior of some patients in both categories may be characterized by deficiencies in control processes relevant to goal determination.

This overlap in underlying cognitive processes may explain why compulsive and impulsive events at first appear phenomenologically distinct but nevertheless may have certain similarities. For example, impairment in goal determination may account for why some compulsive patients finally reach their decisions with unexpected suddenness, in a way that is redolent of impulsive patients with impaired ability to evaluate consequences. Similarly, impairment in goal determination with perseverative response sets in some patients in both categories would lead to similar difficulties on neuropsychological tests of frontal lobe executive function.

On the other hand, certain cognitive structures and processes in compulsivity and impulsivity may be entirely distinct. The structures that mediate grooming and aggressive behaviors are rather different. Similarly, the kind of distortion that is characteristic of some patients in each category may be dissimilar, with exaggerated harm assessment in compulsivity and diminished harm assessment in impulsivity. Information processing in OCD may at times overemphasize internal cues, whereas information processing in impulsive aggression may at times overemphasize immediate external cues. These differences may lead to entirely different responses on the same psychobiological measure (Hollander et al. 1994).

# Conclusions

There are immediate advantages and disadvantages to the cognitive science perspective of compulsivity and impulsivity described in this chapter. One advantage is that cognitive science is a multidisciplinary field that permits incorporation of several different kinds of information and therefore provides an extension beyond strictly biological approaches. Cognitive science also employs methodologies and constructs that are at the cutting edge of the contemporary psychological sciences (H. Gardner 1985; Posner 1990), perhaps giving its proponents an advantage over those who remain constrained to a more traditional psychoanalytic approach.

It may be countered that there are cognitive scientists who are interested purely in the cognitive level of information processing and who ignore all considerations about the medium (e.g., silicon, plasma) in which information processing takes place. Nevertheless, neuroscience can also be understood as constituting an important lower limiting level for cognitive science. This is the path taken in the framework presented here. It is clear, for example, that OCD and impulsive aggression are not simply genetic disorders, in the way that eye color is genetically determined. On the other hand, the neurobiological basis of cognitive structures and processes should not be ignored. Similarly, anthropological and social studies can be understood as constituting an upper limiting level for cognitive science. Although we have not focused on this level, research here may be particularly relevant to impulsive aggressive structures and processes and should be included in clinical evaluation and intervention.

Limitations of the cognitivist view do, however, include the methodological problems posed by the measurement of the posited structures and processes. In the cognitive psychopathology literature, for example, it has been pointed out that self-administered questionnaires do not address underlying cognitive structures (Segal 1988). On the other hand, the use of more sophisticated methodologies (such as those described in Horowitz 1991) may ultimately prove productive in allowing the investigation of cognitive structures and processes in the clinical setting. At present, however, there is a relative paucity of data about cognitive aspects of both compulsivity (Reed 1991) and impulsivity (Barratt 1987).

Conversely, the focus of cognitive science models on discrete structures and processes may come about at the expense of a loss of descriptive and explanatory detail. Freud and subsequent psychoanalysts have often succeeded in providing detailed accounts of underlying psychic structures while retaining the complexity of clinical phenomena. A cognitive science approach to compulsivity and impulsivity must ultimately meet this challenge, tackling such complex subjects and subjectivities as guilt, conscience, and so on. This will require further detailed study of structures such as schemas of self and others in compulsive and impulsive patients.

The field of cognitive clinical science is a growing one, and it offers the potential for providing the clinician with an important integrative perspective (Stein 1994; Stein and Young 1992). Conversely, the clinic can provide cognitive scientists with a rich range of phenomena that, taken together, provide a more comprehensive picture of human cognitive functioning. For example, in this chapter, the automaticity of cognitive processes in both compulsivity and impulsivity was noted. Relatively little is known by cognitive scientists about the control of cognitive processes (Logan and Cowan 1984); clinical science may shed significant light on this and related subjects.

# References

Baer L, Minichiello WE: Behavior therapy for obsessive-compulsive disorder, in Obsessive-Compulsive Disorders: Theory and Management, 2nd Edition. Edited by Jenike MA, Baer L, Minichiello WE. Chicago, IL, Year Book Medical, 1990, pp 203–232

Barratt ES: Impulsiveness and anxiety: information processing and electroencephalograph topography. Journal of Research in Personality 21:453–463, 1987

Bear DM: Neurological perspectives on aggression. J Neuropsychiatry Clin Neurosci 3 (suppl 1):3–8, 1991

Beck AT: Depression: Clinical, Experimental, and Theoretical Aspects. New York, Harper & Row, 1967

Brunner HG, Nelen M, Breakefield XO, et al: Abnormal behavior associated with a point mutation in the structural gene for monoamine oxidase A. Science 262:578–580, 1993

Depue RA, Spoont MR: Conceptualizing a serotonin trait: a behavioral dimension of constraint, in Psychobiology of Suicidal Behavior. Edited by Mann JJ, Stanley M. New York, New York Academy of Sciences, 1987, pp 47–62

Ellis A: Reason and Emotion in Psychotherapy. Secaucus, NJ, Lyle Stuart and Citadel Press, 1962

Ferguson TJ, Rule BG: An attributional perspective on anger and aggression, in Aggression: Theoretical and Empirical Reviews, Vol 1. Edited by Green RG, Donnerstein EI. New York, Academic Press, 1983, pp 41–74

Forgas JP: Cognitive representations of aggression, in Violent Transactions: The Limits of Personality. Edited by Campbell A, Gibbs J. Oxford, UK, Blackwell Scientific, 1986

Freud S: Notes upon a case of obsessional neurosis (1909), in Standard Edition of the Complete Psychological Works of Sigmund Freud, Vol 10. Translated and edited by Strachey J. London, Hogarth Press, 1955, pp 151–318

Freud S: The disposition to obsessional neurosis (1913), in Standard Edition of the Complete Psychological Works of Sigmund Freud, Vol 12. Translated and edited by Strachey J. London, Hogarth Press, 1958, pp 311–326

Freud S: Inhibitions, symptoms and anxiety (1926), in Standard Edition of the Complete Psychological Works of Sigmund Freud, Vol 20. Translated and edited by Strachey J. London, Hogarth Press, 1959, pp 75–175

Gardner H: The Mind's New Science. New York, Basic Books, 1985

Gardner RW, Holzman PS, Klein GS, et al: Cognitive control: a study of individual consistencies in cognitive behavior. Psychological Issues 1:1–185, 1959

Goldstein A, Carr E, Davidson W, et al: In Response to Aggression: Methods of Control and Prosocial Alternatives. New York, Pergamon, 1979

Gorenstein EE: A cognitive perspective on antisocial personality, in Cognitive Bases of Mental Disorders. Edited by Magaro PA. Newbury Park, CA, Sage, 1991, pp 100–133

Hains AA, Ryan EB: The development of social cognitive processes among juvenile delinquents and nondelinquent peers. Child Dev 54:1536–1544, 1983

Head D, Bolton D, Hymas N: Deficit in cognitive shifting ability in patients with obsessive-compulsive disorder. Biol Psychiatry 25:929–937, 1989

Hollander E, Schiffman E, Cohen B, et al: Signs of central nervous system dysfunction in obsessive-compulsive disorder. Arch Gen Psychiatry 47:27–32, 1990

Hollander E, DeCaria CM, Sauoud J, et al: Neurological soft signs in obsessive-compulsive disorder. Arch Gen Psychiatry 48:278–279, 1991

Hollander E, Stein DJ, DeCaria CM: Impulsivity and compulsivity: symptoms and diagnoses. International Psychiatry Today 1:11–12, 1993

Hollander E, Stein DJ, DeCaria CM, et al: Serotonergic sensitivity in borderline personality disorder: preliminary findings. Am J Psychiatry 151:277–280, 1994

Horowitz MJ: A model of mourning: change in schemas of self and other. J Am Psychoanal Assoc 37:297–324, 1989

Horowitz MJ: Person Schemas and Maladaptive Interpersonal Behavior Patterns. Chicago, IL, University of Chicago Press, 1991

Huesman LR: An information processing model for the development of aggression. Aggressive Behavior 14:13–24, 1988

Ingram RE, Kendall PC: Cognitive clinical psychology: implications of an information-processing perspective, in Information Processing Approaches to Clinical Psychology. Edited by Ingram RE. New York, Academic Press, 1986, pp 1–21

Insel TR: Towards a neuroanatomy of obsessive-compulsive disorder. Arch Gen Psychiatry 49:739–744, 1992

Kagan J: The Second Year: The Emergence of Self-Awareness. Cambridge, MA, Harvard University Press, 1981

Kandel E, Freed D: Frontal-lobe dysfunction and antisocial behavior: a review. J Clin Psychol 45:404–413, 1989

Kendall PC, Braswell L: Cognitive-Behavioral Therapy for Impulsive Children, 2nd Edition. New York, Guilford, 1993

Klein GS: Need and regulation. Nebr Symp Motiv, 1954, pp 224–274

Lakoff G: Women, Fire, and Dangerous Things: What Categories Reveal About the Mind. Chicago, IL, University of Chicago Press, 1987

Linehan MM: Cognitive-Behavioral Treatment of Borderline Personality Disorder. New York, Guilford, 1993

Logan GD, Cowan WB: On the ability to inhibit thought and action: a theory of an act of control. Psychol Rev 3:295–327, 1984

Martin LL, Tesser A: Toward a motivational and structural theory of ruminative thought, in Unintended Thought. Edited by Uleman JS, Bargh JA. New York, Guilford, 1989, pp 306–326

Meichenbaum D, Butler L: Cognitive ethology: assessing the streams of cognition and emotion, in Advances in the Study of Communication, Vol 6. Edited by Blankenstein KR, Pliner P, Polivy J. New York, Plenum, 1980

Messer SB: Reflection-impulsivity: a review: Psychol Bull 83:1026–1052, 1976

Messer SB, Schacht TE: A cognitive-dynamic theory of reflection-impulsivity, in Empirical Studies of Psychoanalytic Theory. Edited by Masling J. Hillsdale, NJ, Lawrence Erlbaum, 1986, pp 151–195

Miller L: Neurocognitive Aspects of Remorse: Impulsivity-Compulsivity-Reflectivity. New York, Haworth Press, 1989

Nasby W, Kihlstrom JF: Cognitive assessment of personality and psychopathology, in Information Processing Approaches to Clinical Psychology. Edited by Ingram RE. New York, Academic Press, 1986, pp 219–240

Newman JP, Wallace JF: Psychopathy and cognition, in Psychopathology and Cognition. Edited by Dobson KS, Kendall PC. San Diego, CA, Academic Press, 1993, pp 293–345

Neziroglu F, Anemone R, Yaryura-Tobias JA: Onset of obsessive-compulsive disorder in pregnancy. Am J Psychiatry 149:947–950, 1992

Novaco RW: Anger Control: The Development and Evaluation of an Experimental Treatment. Lexington, MA, DC Heath, 1975

Novaco RW, Welsh WN: Anger disturbances: cognitive mediation and clinical prescriptions, in Clinical Approaches to Violence. Edited by Howells K, Hollin CR. New York, Wiley, 1989, pp 39–60

Peterfreund E: Information, Systems and Psychoanalysis: An Evolutionary Biological Approach to Psychoanalytic Theory. New York, International Universities Press, 1971

Posner MI (ed): Foundations of Cognitive Science. Cambridge, MA, The MIT Press, 1990

Rapoport JL, Ryland DH, Kriete M: Drug treatment of canine acral lick: an animal model of obsessive-compulsive disorder. Arch Gen Psychiatry 49:517–521, 1992

Reed G: The cognitive characteristics of obsessional disorder, in Cognitive Biases of Mental Disorders. Edited by Magaro PA. Newbury Park, CA, Sage, 1991, pp 77–99

Rumelhart DE, Hinton GE, PDP Research Group (eds): Parallel Distributed Processing: Explorations in the Microstructure of Cognition. Cambridge, MA, The MIT Press, 1986

Salkovskis PM, Warwick HMC: Cognitive therapy of obsessive-compulsive disorder, in The Theory and Practice of Cognitive Therapy. Edited by Perris C, Blackburn IM, Perris H. Heidelberg, Springer, 1988

118     *Impulsivity and Compulsivity*

Segal ZV: Appraisal of the self-schemata construct in cognitive models of depression. Psychol Bull 103:147–162, 1988

Stein DJ: Psychoanalysis and cognitive science: contrasting models of the mind. J Am Acad Psychoanal 20:543–559, 1992a

Stein DJ: Schemas in the cognitive and clinical sciences: an integrative construct. Journal of Psychotherapy Integration 2:45–63, 1992b

Stein DJ: Cognitive science and psychiatry: an overview. Integrative Psychiatry 9:13–24, 1994

Stein DJ, Hollander E: Cognitive science and obsessive-compulsive disorder, in Cognitive Science and Clinical Disorders. Edited by Stein DJ, Young JE. San Diego, CA, Academic Press, 1992, pp 1–17

Stein DJ, Hollander E: Impulsive aggression and obsessive-compulsive disorder. Psychiatric Annals 23:389–395, 1993

Stein DJ, Young JE (eds): Cognitive Science and Clinical Disorders. New York, Academic Press, 1992

Stein DJ, Shoulberg N, Helton K, et al: A neuroethological model of OCD. Compr Psychiatry 33:274–281, 1992

Stein DJ, Hollander E, Chan S, et al: Computerized tomography and soft signs in obsessive-compulsive disorder. Psychiatry Res 50:143–150, 1993a

Stein DJ, Hollander E, Cohen L, et al: Neuropsychiatric impairment in impulsive personality disorders. Psychiatry Res 48:257–266, 1993b

Stein DJ, Hollander E, Liebowitz MR: Neurobiology of impulsivity and impulse control disorders. J Neuropsychiatry Clin Neurosci 5:9–17, 1993c

Stein DJ, Hollander E, Simeon D, et al: Pregnancy and obsessive-compulsive disorder (letter). Am J Psychiatry 150:1131–1132, 1993d

Stein DJ, Hollander E, Cohen L: Neuropsychiatry of OCD, in The First International Conference on Obsessive-Compulsive Disorder. Edited by Hollander E, Marazziti D, Zohar J. New York, Wiley, 1994, pp 167–182

Stein DJ, Hollander E, Towey J: Neuropsychiatry of impulsivity and aggression, in Impulsivity and Aggression. Edited by Hollander E, Stein DJ. New York, Wiley, 1995, pp 91–108

Thorndyke PW, Hayes-Roth B: The use of schemata in the acquisition and transference of knowledge. Cognitive Psychology 11:82–106, 1979

Towey J, Bruder G, Hollander E, et al: Endogenous event-related potentials in obsessive-compulsive disorder. Biol Psychiatry 28:92–98, 1990

Zohar J, Insel TR: Obsessive-compulsive disorder: psychobiological approaches to diagnosis, treatment, and pathophysiology. Biol Psychiatry 22:667–687, 1987

# 5

# Biology and Pharmacological Treatment of Impulse-Control Disorders

Richard J. Kavoussi, M.D.
Emil F. Coccaro, M.D.

---

Impulsive behavior disorders are a source of distress and frustration to patients, their families, and the clinicians who work with them. The major psychiatric disorders of impulse control (kleptomania, pathological gambling, trichotillomania, pyromania, etc.) involve a failure to resist an impulse to behave in some way that is harmful to the individual or others, an increasing sense of arousal or tension before committing/engaging in the act, and an experience of pleasure, gratification, or release of tension at the time of committing the act. Some other major psychiatric syndromes such as the paraphilias, bulimia, and substance use disorders also involve an inability to resist harmful impulses, a sense of arousal or tension before engaging in the pathological behavior, and the experience of pleasure and release of tension afterward.

In contrast to the episodic loss of impulse control found in the major psychiatric disorders noted above, chronic aggressive or impulsive behavior is characteristic of individuals with certain personality disorders (e.g., borderline, antisocial). Many of these individuals exhibit lifelong problems with impulsive aggressive behavior, either acting out against others or inflicting harm on themselves.

It is not clear whether impulsive behavior disorders are simple variants of compulsive behavior disorders (e.g., obsessive-compulsive disorder [OCD]) or are on the opposite end of the behavioral spectrum. Both impulsive and compulsive disorders involve a failure to resist a drive to act in a way that is potentially self-damaging, escalation of anxiety before engaging in the act, and relief of anxiety following the act. In fact, one of the few differences between the two types of disorders is that most compulsive behavior disorders are perceived by the patient as ego-dystonic, whereas impulsive behaviors are viewed as usually ego-syntonic. Rather than being the dimensional opposite of obsessive-compulsive disorders, impulse-control disorders (both major disorders and personality disorders with significant impulsivity) may represent a different phenomenological manifestation of a group of disorders sharing the feature of decreased ability to inhibit motor responses to affective states. In fact, phenomenological and family studies suggest a strong relationship between affective, anxiety, obsessive, and impulsive behavior disorders (Apter et al. 1990; McElroy et al. 1992).

In this chapter we review current knowledge concerning biological and pharmacological treatment findings in patients with impulse-control disorders. In this process we explore whether impulse-control disorders share biological and treatment features similar to or different from those found in OCD.

## Biology of Impulsive Disorders

Biological studies of individuals with impulse-control disorders have repeatedly suggested a relationship between central nervous system (CNS) catecholamine function and impulsive behaviors. The major transmitter systems involved in regulating impulsivity appear to be the serotonergic system (involving serotonin [5-hydroxytryptamine; 5-HT]), the noradrenergic system (involving norepinephrine), and the dopaminergic system (involving dopamine). As discussed below, impaired brain serotonin function and hyperactive norepinephrine/dopamine function appear to be correlated with increased risk of impulsive behavior.

## Serotonergic System Function and Impulsive Behavior

Animal studies have repeatedly shown an inverse relationship between impulsive aggressive responses and central serotonergic system function. For example, shock-induced fighting in rats was found to be potentiated by pretreatment with the serotonergic neuron toxin 5,7-dihydroxytryptamine (Kantak et al. 1981). Conversely, 5-hydroxytryptophan (a serotonin precursor) was found to reverse aggressive behavior associated with lesions of serotonergic neurons in rats (Dichiara et al. 1971). Mouse killing behavior following pretreatment with p-chlorophenylalanine (a serotonin neurotoxin) is blocked by the serotonin reuptake inhibitor fluoxetine (Berzenyi et al. 1983). Finally, a strong negative correlation was found between aggression and cerebrospinal fluid (CSF) concentrations of 5-hydroxyindoleacetic acid (5-HIAA), the major metabolite of serotonin, in free-ranging rhesus monkeys (Mehlman et al. 1994).

Assessments of CNS serotonin function in humans also repeatedly demonstrate an inverse correlation with impulsive aggressive behavior. Åsberg and colleagues (1976) demonstrated an association between reduced CSF 5-HIAA and violent suicidal behavior in depressed patients. G. L. Brown and co-workers (1979) found an inverse relationship between life history of physical aggression and CSF 5-HIAA concentration in military recruits with DSM-II–defined personality disorders. Many subsequent studies have reported inverse correlations between CSF 5-HIAA concentration and impulsive behavior in humans, regardless of specific psychiatric diagnosis (G. L. Brown and Linnoila 1990; Coccaro et al. 1989b). Violent suicide attempters show lower CSF levels of 5-HIAA than nonviolent suicide attempters (Träskman-Bendz et al. 1992). Depressed patients with reduced CSF 5-HIAA concentration show not only an increased rate of suicide attempts but also an increased frequency of outward-directed aggression (van Praag 1986). Violent offenders with a history of serious suicide attempts were found to have reduced CSF 5-HIAA concentrations compared with similar offenders without a history of serious suicidal behavior (Virkkunen et al. 1989). Reduced CSF 5-HIAA concentration in these individuals was also associated with future violent acts during a 3-year follow-up period. CSF 5-HIAA concentrations measured in children and adolescents with disruptive behavior disorders have been found to be inversely correlated with measures of aggression (Kruesi et al. 1990). CSF 5-HIAA concentration has also been found to be inversely correlated with history of cruelty to animals in children (Kruesi 1989).

Reduced CSF 5-HIAA concentration correlates with impulsive rather than premeditated aggression (Linnoila et al. 1983). For example, impulsive fire setters have lower CSF 5-HIAA concentrations than fire setters who also engage in other, nonimpulsive antisocial acts (Virkkunen et al. 1987). This finding suggests that abnormalities in the brain's serotonergic system functioning predispose individuals to impulsive aggressive behaviors rather than to nonimpulsive aggressive behaviors.

Pharmacochallenge studies examine the neuroendocrine response to an acute challenge with an agent that acts on a specific central neurotransmitter system. One advantage of this method is that the outcome measures reflect dynamic functioning of central neurotransmitter systems in specific brain areas (e.g., within the limbic-hypothalamic-pituitary axis). These studies, like the studies described above, demonstrate evidence of a relationship between decreased central serotonergic system function and impulsive aggression in humans. For example, fenfluramine is a medication that releases serotonin from presynaptic neurons. This increase in central serotonin usually results in a transient but marked increase in serum prolactin. There is a strong inverse relationship between the prolactin response to fenfluramine challenge and indices of irritable, impulsive aggression in male personality disorder patients regardless of the particular personality disorder (Coccaro et al. 1989b). In other words, patients with high degrees of lifelong irritability and impulsive aggression have a lower or blunted prolactin response to fenfluramine compared with healthy control subjects. Other studies have consistently found an inverse relationship between indices of central serotonergic system function and impulsive aggression in patients with mood and personality disorders with various challenge agents, such as fenfluramine (DeMeo et al. 1989), the direct serotonin receptor agonist $m$-chlorophenylpiperazine (m-CPP) (Coccaro et al. 1989a; Hollander et al. 1994; Moss et al. 1990), and the 5-HT$_{1A}$ agonist buspirone (Coccaro et al. 1990b).

Other measures of central serotonergic system function are abnormal in patients with a history of aggressive behavior. For example, tritiated imipramine binding (a measure of presynaptic serotonin function) was found to be reduced in the brains of violent suicide victims (Stanley et al. 1982). Conversely, increased postsynaptic 5-HT$_2$ receptor binding has been found in the prefrontal cortex of the brains of suicide victims (Arango et al. 1990; Mann et al. 1986), especially those who had used violent methods (Arora and Meltzer 1989). Measures of serotonin platelet uptake correlate inversely with measures of impulsivity in male patients with episodic aggression (C. S. Brown et al. 1989). In addition, serotonin platelet uptake was found to be reduced in impulsive alcohol abusers compared with control subjects (Bailly et al. 1990).

Subtypes of serotonin receptors may differentially mediate impulsive aggressive behaviors. For example, animal studies suggest that 5-HT$_{1A}$ receptor stimulation results in a decrease in aggressive behavior (Beckett et al. 1992). Similarly, aggressive personality disorder patients show a blunted prolactin response to the 5-HT$_{1A}$ agonist buspirone (Coccaro et al. 1990b).

Finally, there is preliminary evidence for a genetic disturbance predisposing individuals to impulsive aggressive behavior. Reduced central serotonergic system function in personality disorder patients was found to be correlated with an increased risk of impulsivity in their first-degree relatives (Coccaro et al. 1994).

Recently, a portion of the gene for tryptophan hydroxylase (the rate-limiting enzyme for serotonin synthesis) has been discovered to exist as at least two alleles: U and L. Investigation in human subjects has suggested that presence of either the UL or the LL genotype is associated with impulsive aggressive and suicidal behavior and low levels of CSF 5-HIAA in violent offenders (Nielsen et al. 1994).

## Noradrenergic and Dopaminergic System Function and Impulsive Behavior

Although the serotonergic system has been the most widely studied neurotransmitter system in relation to impulsivity, there is strong evidence for a role of the dopaminergic and noradrenergic systems in the genesis of impulsive behavior. Animal studies suggest that increases in dopamine activity create a state in which animals are more prepared to respond impulsively to stimuli in the environment (Blackburn et al. 1992). Antidepressants that inhibit noradrenergic uptake or stimulate noradrenergic output have been found to increase aggressive behavior in isolated mice (Cai et al. 1993). In addition, CSF norepinephrine concentrations were found to be positively correlated with high rankings of aggression in free-ranging rhesus monkeys (Higley et al. 1992).

Hyperactivity of noradrenergic functioning has been found to correlate with disorders of impulse control in humans as well. Increased beta-noradrenergic receptor binding in the prefrontal and temporal cortices in the brains of suicide victims compared with accident victims has been reported in many studies (Arango et al. 1990; Biegon and Israeli 1988; Mann et al. 1986). Conversely, reduced alpha₁-noradrenergic receptor binding has been found in the prefrontal and temporal cortices and in the caudate nucleus of brains of suicide victims (Gross-Isseroff et al. 1990).

Elevated CSF MHPG (3-methoxy-4-hydroxyphenylglycol), the primary metabolite of central norepinephrine, and urinary norepinephrine concentrations were reported in pathological gamblers who were compared with healthy volunteers (Roy et al. 1988). Strong positive correlations were also noted between these indices of central noradrenergic system function and indices of "extroversion" (Roy et al. 1989). These findings suggest that an abnormality in central noradrenergic system function may underlie the "sensation seeking" characteristic of the compulsive gambler. Similarly, in one study, urinary norepinephrine concentrations were found to be higher in depressed patients with a history of suicidal behavior compared with those without such a history; elevated urinary norepinephrine was also positively correlated with low suicide intent (i.e., impulsivity) (Mancini and Brown 1992). CSF MHPG levels are elevated in violent suicide attempters compared with nonviolent suicide attempters (Träskman-Bendz et al. 1992). In one study (Coccaro et al. 1991), growth hormone responses to the alpha$_2$-noradrenergic receptor agonist clonidine were found to be significantly greater in personality disorder patients than in remitted depressive patients or healthy control subjects. These responses correlated positively with self-report measures of lifetime irritability (but not assaultiveness) in both the personality disorder patients and the healthy control subjects.

# Pharmacological Treatment of Impulsive Disorders

Most of the published literature concerning the medication management of impulse-control disorders consists of uncontrolled case studies. From the discussion of the biology of impulsive behavior in the previous section, it would be expected that medications that enhance serotonergic functioning or decrease noradrenergic/dopaminergic functioning would be most helpful in reducing impulsive behavior. Thus, medications that might be effective include dopamine blocking agents (neuroleptics), antimanic agents (lithium, carbamazepine, valproate), beta-noradrenergic receptor antagonists, and serotonin reuptake inhibitors and agonists.

## Medications

### Dopamine Blocking Agents

Antipsychotic agents are often used to treat impulsive aggressive behavior. However, it is not clear whether the antiaggressive effects of these agents are related to dopaminergic blockade or to non-specific sedation. Open-label thioridazine has been reported to diminish impulsive behavior in patients with borderline personality disorder (Teicher et al. 1989). Similarly, in a large sample of patients with borderline and/or schizotypal personality disorder, treatment with low-dose haloperidol was associated with significant improvement in ratings of hostility and impulsivity compared with amitriptyline or placebo (Soloff et al. 1989). However, these findings were not reproduced in two other double-blind, placebo-controlled studies of borderline and schizotypal personality disorder patients who were treated with thiothixene (Goldberg et al. 1986) or trifluoperazine (Cowdry and Gardner 1988). On the other hand, in a placebo-controlled study of personality disorder patients with a history of multiple impulsive suicide attempts, the neuroleptic flupentixol significantly reduced suicidal behavior (Montgomery and Montgomery 1982). These findings suggest that low-dose dopamine blocking agents may be effective treatments for selected patients with impulse-control disorders. Unfortunately, the risk of extrapyramidal side effects and tardive dyskinesia warrants caution in the indiscriminate use of these medications.

### Noradrenergic Blocking Agents

Beta-adrenergic receptor antagonists have been used to treat aggressive behavior in certain psychiatric populations in several uncontrolled studies. High doses of beta-blockers (e.g., propranolol, nadolol) may decrease aggressive behavior in various patients with chronic organic brain syndromes (Yudofsky et al. 1981), chronic psychiatric inpatients (Ratey et al. 1992), patients with schizophrenia (Sorgi et al. 1986), or adults with temper outbursts and residual attention-deficit disorder (Mattes 1986). Further controlled studies of beta-adrenergic and alpha-adrenergic blockers are needed in patients with impulse-control disorders to determine their full range of efficacy.

### Antimanic Agents

Medications used to treat mania reduce affective lability and thus may reduce behavioral lability as well.

Some studies suggest that lithium carbonate may be of value in the treatment of patients with impulse-control disorders. Lithium was found to be more effective than placebo in reducing mood lability in patients with "emotionally unstable character disorder" (Rifkin et al. 1972), a group of patients characterized by intense, rapidly shifting affects and impulse-control problems. Lithium has been reported to reduce impulsive aggression in prison inmates in both open (Tupin et al. 1973) and blinded placebo-controlled trials (Sheard et al. 1976) and in blinded placebo-controlled trials in hospitalized children with conduct disorder (Campbell et al. 1984). Case reports also suggest the efficacy of lithium in specific impulse-control disorders such as trichotillomania (Christenson et al. 1991).

Carbamazepine, an anticonvulsant, is another antimanic agent that may be effective in the treatment of impulse-control disorders. Open-label trials with carbamazepine suggest that this agent may be effective in reducing self-destructive behavior in mental retardation (Winchel and Stanley 1991) and in reducing aggression in children with conduct disorder (Kafantaris et al. 1992). One blinded, placebo-controlled trial found carbamazepine to be the only agent that selectively decreased behavioral outbursts in patients with borderline personality disorder (Cowdry and Gardner 1988). Valproic acid, another anticonvulsant used in the treatment of mania, may also prove to be effective in the treatment of impulsive aggression (Mattes 1992).

Although the exact mechanism of action is unclear, carbamazepine has been reported to increase plasma levels of the serotonin precursor tryptophan (Pratt et al. 1984) and to increase the prolactin response to tryptophan challenge (Elphick et al. 1990). These findings raise the possibility that antimanic agents enhance central serotonergic system functioning and thus decrease biological vulnerability to impulsive behavior.

**Serotonergic Agents**

Antidepressant medications have been investigated as treatments for impulsivity and aggression because of their ability to enhance serotonergic system functioning. Unfortunately, tricyclic antidepressants have been associated with increased impulse-control problems in subgroups of personality disorder patients who are prone to impulsivity (Soloff et al. 1986). In one double-blind study (Soloff et al. 1986), amitriptyline was generally less effective than haloperidol, and almost half of the patients who were treated with amitriptyline had more acting-out behavior than at baseline. In another double-blind study, desipramine was no better than placebo in reducing impulsive aggressive behavior in patients with borderline personality disorder (Links et al. 1990). These poor results may be due to the fact that these medications increase noradrenergic system functioning along with serotonergic system functioning, thus sometimes leading to a paradoxical increase in impulsive aggressive behavior.

Monoamine oxidase inhibitors (MAOIs) also yield variable therapeutic results in patients with impulse-control disorders. Improvement in mood was reported in one study of patients with borderline personality disorder who were treated with tranylcypromine compared with treatment with carbamazepine, trifluoperazine, alprazolam, or placebo (Cowdry and Gardner 1988). Improvement in impulse control, however, was only apparent on self-report ratings. A greater global response was reported for phenelzine compared with imipramine in a study of patients with atypical depression and borderline personality disorder (Parsons et al. 1989). On the other hand, another study reported only modest benefits of MAOIs in borderline patients (Cornelius et al. 1991). Again, the fact that these medications increase both serotonergic and noradrenergic system functioning may reduce their effectiveness in this population.

The effect of medication that specifically enhances serotonergic system functioning on impulse-control problems has, despite a compelling rationale, received only limited study to date. Open treatment with 5-hydroxytryptophan in self-injuring patients with Lesch-Nyhan syndrome decreased self-injurious behavior in one report (Mizuno and Yugari 1974). A self-injuring patient with major depression responded to trazodone (Patel et al. 1988), a medication with both serotonin agonist and antagonistic properties. The serotonin reuptake inhibitor clomipramine was effective in reducing hair-pulling behavior in patients with trichotillomania in an open trial (Pollard et al. 1991) and was more effective than desipramine in a double-blind study (Swedo et al. 1989). Serotonin reuptake inhibitors have also been found to be helpful in reducing sexual obsessions and, to a lesser degree, paraphilias (Stein et al. 1992). Clomipramine was found to be effective in treating compulsive gambling in at least one case report (Hollander et al. 1992b).

Studies of serotonergic agents in patients with impulsive personality disorders are only in their beginning stages. The selective serotonin reuptake inhibitor fluoxetine has been generally effective during open treatment in some patients with borderline personality disorder, particularly those without depression (Norden 1989). Similar responses to fluoxetine in borderline personality disorder have been reported in inpatients, particularly in regard to suicidal ideation and impulse-control problems (Cornelius et al. 1991). In one report (Coccaro et al. 1990a), fluoxetine treatment was associated with substantial reductions in overt aggressive behavior and irritability in three nondepressed personality disorder outpatients with histories of prominent impulsive aggressive behavior. In an open clinical trial, the serotonin uptake inhibitor sertraline was found to be effective in reducing impulsive aggressive behavior in a group of 11 patients with a variety of personality disorders (Kavoussi et al. 1994). Other serotonin reuptake inhibitors (e.g., paroxetine, fluvoxamine) may also prove effective for these patients.

Serotonin$_{1A}$ agonists may be particularly effective in reducing impulsive behavior problems. For example, buspirone, a 5-HT$_{1A}$ partial agonist, appears to be helpful in reducing aggression in mentally retarded patients (Ratey et al. 1991). Further studies need to examine the role of other 5-HT$_{1A}$ agents (e.g., gepirone, ipsapirone, flesinoxan) in the treatment of impulsive aggressive behavior.

Unfortunately, there have not been any published long-term follow-up studies of impulsive patients treated with serotonergic agents. Such studies are necessary to determine whether initial response to medications continues with long-term treatment. In a group of 15 personality disorder patients who remained on open fluoxetine following a 3-month double-blind study (follow-up 3 to 18 months), there was no return to pretreatment levels of impulsive aggression (R. J. Kavoussi and E. F. Coccaro, unpublished data, 1996).

Although the above discussion strongly suggests that enhancing serotonergic activity and decreasing noradrenergic activity are the keys to reducing impulsive aggressive behavior in many patients, there are other agents that seem to be effective in reducing impulsivity in individual patients. Patients with residual attention-deficit disorder may exhibit impulsive aggressive behavior (Wender et al. 1981). These patients may benefit from treatment with noradrenergic enhancing agents such as stimulants or bupropion (Wender and Reimherr 1990). Opiate antagonists have been used to treat patients with developmental disabilities and self-injurious behavior, which suggests a role for the endogenous opiate system in the pathogenesis of such behavior (Herman et al. 1987). Future studies will be needed to help us determine which treatment is best suited for each patient.

## Clinical Vignettes

The following cases illustrate the typical presentation of patients with impulsive disorders and their response to treatment.

■ Vignette 1

Ms. A., a 27-year-old woman, presented for treatment at the insistence of her husband. The patient admitted to frequent violent arguments with her husband, family, co-workers, and, often, strangers. She had lost many jobs because of her mood lability and intense, inappropriate anger. She was also violent with her husband during arguments over seemingly trivial matters. For example, Ms. A. hit her husband's head against the steering column when he became lost on the way to a movie theater. She had gotten into similarly violent arguments with her sister and mother and was losing her temper with her 3-year-old daughter, slapping her on several occasions. Ms. A. would usually feel guilty after these events and had attempted suicide several times. Previous treatment with supportive psychotherapy had been unsuccessful. The patient was begun on fluoxetine 20 mg/day. After 5 weeks of treatment, Ms. A. noted a marked decrease in her irritability. She had a dramatic decrease in temper outbursts and was able to "lose my temper without losing control."

■ Vignette 2

Mr. B., a 33-year-old man, was brought to the clinic by his wife. She complained that he was self-centered and had a violent temper. He often slapped her during arguments and threw furniture around their home when arguing with her. He worked in a responsible position in a local hospital but had been unable to continue in jobs for long because of inappropriate anger at little provocation. Mr. B. had tried to commit suicide once in the past. Although he acknowledged problems in his relationships and at work, he tended to blame others for "purposely doing things they know will get me angry." He began treatment with sertraline 50 mg/day, increasing to 100 mg/day after 2 weeks. Although he noted no real change at first, his wife reported a marked decrease in his aggressive behavior and irritability after 4 weeks of treatment. However, Mr. B. stopped the medication on his own after 8 weeks of treatment and returned to his baseline level of irritability and aggressive behavior. He restarted sertraline 100 mg/day at the insistence of his wife, and after 2 weeks a decrease in impulsive aggression was again noted. After stopping and restarting sertraline one more time with similar results, Mr. B. admitted that he might benefit from continued treatment with medication.

## Comparison of Impulsive and
## Compulsive Behavior Disorders

### Biology

Both impulsive and compulsive behavior disorders appear to involve disruptions in serotonergic neurotransmitter function. We have reviewed the evidence for decreased serotonin function in impulsive behavior disorders. There is accumulating evidence that serotonin abnormalities also underlie the symptoms of compulsive disorders such as OCD (Barr et al. 1992). Some studies suggest that compulsive behavior disorders such as OCD involve increased sensitivity of serotonin receptors. This would imply that impulsive and compulsive behavior disorders are on opposite ends of a biological and behavioral spectrum. For example, an increase in platelet serotonin uptake in OCD patients compared with control subjects suggests an increase in serotonergic activity in these patients (Vitiello et al. 1991). In one study, obsessive symptoms in patients with Tourette's disorder were related to higher levels of 5-HIAA and to a higher turnover of serotonin (Bornstein and Baker 1992). In another study, OCD patients who received pretreatment with the serotonin receptor blocker metergoline before m-CPP challenge experienced no significant changes from baseline OCD symptoms or other behavioral changes; the ability of m-CPP to elicit elevations in plasma prolactin was also blocked by metergoline pretreatment (Pigott et al. 1991).

On the other hand, many studies suggest a decrease in serotonergic functioning in OCD. This would suggest a biological similarity between impulsive and compulsive disorders. For example, prolactin and cortisol responses to MK-212, a serotonin agonist, were significantly blunted in patients with OCD compared with control subjects, but behavioral ratings were not significantly different in the two groups, suggesting subsensitivity of serotonin receptors in this disorder (Bastani et al. 1990). Platelet imipramine binding and serotonin uptake have been found to be decreased in

OCD patients compared with control subjects (Bastani et al. 1991; Marazziti et al. 1992). Cortisol and prolactin responses to $d$-fenfluramine in nondepressed OCD patients were attenuated compared with the responses in healthy control subjects (Lucey et al. 1992b). Prolactin response appears to be blunted in patients following m-CPP but not following fenfluramine in some studies (Hollander et al. 1992a). In fact, some studies have found no differences between OCD patients and healthy subjects in neuroendocrine responses to serotonergic agents (Charney et al. 1988; McBride et al. 1992).

As in impulse-control disorders, there may be a hypersensitivity of the noradrenergic system in OCD patients. For example, there are increased alpha2-adrenoreceptor binding sites (Lee et al. 1990) and higher levels of platelet sulfotransferase activity (a putative peripheral marker of dopamine function) (Marazziti et al. 1992) in OCD patients compared with control subjects. Similarly, following clonidine, but not following placebo, patients transiently experienced a significant reduction of obsessions and compulsions; however, growth hormone response to clonidine did not differentiate patients from healthy control subjects (Hollander et al. 1991b). These findings lend some support for a derangement of noradrenergic functioning in OCD.

## Psychopharmacological Treatment

As in the impulse-control disorders, medications that enhance serotonin have been helpful in reducing the symptoms of OCD. The selective serotonin reuptake inhibitor fluoxetine and the serotonin reuptake inhibitor clomipramine have been found to be effective agents in the treatment of OCD (Pigott et al. 1990). In a double-blind, random-assignment study, buspirone and clomipramine were found to be equally effective in treating OCD (Pato et al. 1991). Beneficial effects of clomipramine in OCD can be blocked by the serotonin antagonist metergoline, which supports the hypothesis that clomipramine's therapeutic effects in OCD are mediated via serotonergic mechanisms (Benkelfat et al. 1989). The selective serotonin reuptake inhibitor fluvoxamine has been found to be more effective than the norepinephrine uptake inhibitor desipramine in reducing OCD symptoms (Goodman et al. 1990), which again suggests that there is an abnormality in serotonergic functioning in OCD and that effective medications act by inducing adaptive changes in serotonergic receptors. Chronic fluoxetine treatment has been shown to reduce behavioral sensitivity to m-CPP and partially normalize the neuroendocrine response to m-CPP in patients with OCD (Hollander et al. 1991a).

## Conclusions

It is clear that biology and treatment studies of impulse-control disorders share many similarities with biology and treatment studies of OCD. Yet it is still unclear whether impulse-control disorders represent a variant of obsessive behavior disorders or are at the opposite end of the behavioral spectrum. More to the point, why do such disorders, with seemingly disparate clinical presentations, share so many biological abnormalities and respond to treatment in the same way?

One possibility is that these disorders involve abnormalities in different serotonin receptor subsystems. For example, in one study (Lucey et al. 1992a), prolactin responses to the 5-HT$_{1A}$ agonist buspirone were no different in OCD patients and control subjects, which suggests that in OCD a complex interaction of other serotonin receptor subtypes may be occurring, possibly with dysfunction primarily of the 5-HT$_2$ receptors. Similarly, hypothermic and cortisol responses to the 5-HT$_{1A}$ agonist ipsapirone in OCD patients were not significantly different from those in control subjects (Lesch et al. 1991), which again suggests that impulsive and compulsive disorders may involve abnormalities in different subsystems of serotonergic functioning. Unfortunately, studies to date have not demonstrated abnormal 5-HT$_2$ receptor function in platelets of patients with OCD (Pandey et al. 1993).

Another possibility is that impulse-control disorders and obsessive behavior disorders differ in the way various transmitter systems interact. From the data described above, it is clear that a balance between the serotonergic, noradrenergic, and dopaminergic systems exists and that various perturbations of this balance may lead to various forms of psychopathology. For example, impulse-control disorders may involve a pathological decrease in central serotonergic system function that leads to a compensatory increase in noradrenergic functioning and increased acting-out behavior. On the other hand, obsessive behavior disorders might involve abnormal increases in mesocortical dopaminergic functioning and harm avoidance, leading to compensatory changes in serotonergic functioning.

Finally, it is possible that impulse-control disorders and OCD share a common biology but that differences in their clinical presentation are due to differences in environmental factors. For example, abnormalities in serotonergic functioning may lead to an increased vulnerability to rapid and intense affective shifts in response to stress. Early life experiences may lead the individual with this vulnerability to never trust that he or she has completed a task or is safe (as in the case of OCD) or to physically act out as a way of reducing the intensity of affective states (as in the case of impulse-control disorders). If this hypothesis is true, then it is important that psychiatric researchers now turn their attention to the interaction of biological vulnerabilities and learned behaviors in an effort to develop a better understanding of and treatment for our patients.

# References

Apter A, van Praag HM, Plutchik R, et al: Interrelationships among anxiety, aggression, impulsivity, and mood: a serotonergically linked cluster? Psychiatry Res 32:191–199, 1990

Arango V, Ernsberger P, Marzuk PM, et al: Autoradiographic demonstration of increased serotonin 5-HT$_2$ and beta-adrenergic receptor binding sites in the brain of suicide victims. Arch Gen Psychiatry 47: 1038–1047, 1990

Arora RC, Meltzer HY: Serotonergic measures in the brains of suicide victims: 5-HT2 binding sites in the frontal cortex of suicide victims and control subjects. Am J Psychiatry 146:730–736, 1989

Åsberg M, Träskman L, Thorén P: 5-HIAA in the cerebrospinal fluid: a biochemical suicide predictor? Arch Gen Psychiatry 33:1193–1197, 1976

Bailly D, Vignau J, Lauth B, et al: Platelet serotonin decrease in alcoholic patients. Acta Psychiatr Scand 81:68–72, 1990

Barr LC, Goodman WK, Price LH, et al: The serotonin hypothesis of obsessive-compulsive disorder: implications of pharmacologic challenge studies. J Clin Psychiatry 53 (no 4, suppl):17–28, 1992

Bastani B, Nash JF, Meltzer HY: Prolactin and cortisol responses to MK-212, a serotonin agonist, in obsessive-compulsive disorder. Arch Gen Psychiatry 47:833–839, 1990

Bastani B, Arora RC, Meltzer HY: Serotonin uptake and imipramine binding in the blood platelets of obsessive-compulsive disorder patients. Biol Psychiatry 30:131–139, 1991

Beckett SR, Lawrence AJ, Marsden CA, et al: Attenuation of chemically induced defense response by 5-HT1 receptor agonists administered into the periaqueductal gray. Psychopharmacology (Berl) 108:110–114, 1992

Benkelfat C, Murphy DL, Zohar J, et al: Clomipramine in obsessive-compulsive disorder: further evidence for a serotonergic mechanism of action. Arch Gen Psychiatry 46:23–28, 1989

Berzenyi P, Galateo E, Valzelli L: Fluoxetine activity on muricidal aggression induced in rats by p-chlorophenylalanine. Aggressive Behavior 9:333–338, 1983

Biegon A, Israeli M: Regionally selective increases in beta-adrenergic receptor density in brains of suicide victims. Brain Res 442:199–203, 1988

Blackburn JR, Pfaus JG, Phillips AG: Dopamine functions in appetitive and defensive behaviors. Prog Neurobiol 39:247–279, 1992

Bornstein RA, Baker GB: Urinary indoleamines in Tourette syndrome patients with obsessive-compulsive characteristics. Psychiatry Res 41:267–274, 1992

Brown CS, Kent TA, Bryant SG, et al: Blood platelet uptake of serotonin in episodic aggression. Psychiatry Res 27:5–12, 1989

Brown GL, Linnoila MI: CSF serotonin metabolite (5-HIAA) studies in depression, impulsivity, and violence. J Clin Psychiatry 51 (no 4, suppl):31–41, 1990

Brown GL, Goodwin FK, Ballenger JC, et al: Aggression in humans correlates with cerebrospinal fluid metabolite. Psychiatry Res 1:131–139, 1979

Cai B, Matsumoto K, Ohta H, et al: Biphasic effects of typical anti-depressants and mianserin, an atypical antidepressant, on aggressive behavior in socially isolated mice. Pharmacol Biochem Behav 44:519–525, 1993

Campbell M, Small AM, Green WH, et al: Behavioral efficacy of haloperidol and lithium carbonate, a comparison in hospitalized aggressive children with conduct disorder. Arch Gen Psychiatry 41:650–655, 1984

Charney DS, Goodman WK, Price LH, et al: Serotonin function in obsessive-compulsive disorder: a comparison of the effects of tryptophan and m-chlorophenylpiperazine in patients and healthy subjects. Arch Gen Psychiatry 45:177–185, 1988

Christenson GA, Popkin MK, Mackenzie TB, et al: Lithium treatment of chronic hair pulling. J Clin Psychiatry 52:116–120, 1991

Coccaro EF, Siever LJ, Kavoussi RJ, et al: Impulsive aggression in personality disorder: evidence for involvement of 5-HT-1 receptors (abstract). Biol Psychiatry 25:86A, 1989a

Coccaro EF, Siever LJ, Klar HM, et al: Serotonergic studies in affective and personality disorder patients: correlations with behavioral aggression and impulsivity. Arch Gen Psychiatry 46:587–599, 1989b

Coccaro EF, Astill JL, Herbert JL, et al: Fluoxetine treatment of impulsive aggression in DSM-III-R personality disorder patients. J Clin Psychopharmacol 10:373–375, 1990a

Coccaro EF, Gabriel S, Siever LJ: Buspirone challenge: preliminary evidence for a role for central 5HT-1A receptor function in impulsive aggressive behavior in humans. Psychopharmacol Bull 26:393–405, 1990b

Coccaro EF, Lawrence T, Trestman R, et al: Growth hormone responses to intravenous clonidine challenge correlate with behavioral irritability in psychiatric patients and healthy volunteers. Psychiatry Res 39:129–139, 1991

Coccaro EF, Silverman JM, Klar HM, et al: Familial correlates of reduced central serotonergic function in patients with personality disorders. Arch Gen Psychiatry 51:318–324, 1994

Cornelius JR, Soloff PH, Perel JM, et al: A preliminary trial of fluoxetine in refractory borderline patients. J Clin Psychopharmacol 11:116–120, 1991

Cowdry RW, Gardner DL: Pharmacotherapy of borderline personality disorder: alprazolam, carbamazepine, trifluoperazine, and tranylcypromine. Arch Gen Psychiatry 45:111–119, 1988

DeMeo MD, McBride PA, Chen J-S, et al: Relative contribution of MDD and borderline personality disorder to 5-HT responsivity (abstract). Biol Psychiatry 25:85A, 1989

Dichiara G, Camba R, Spano PF: Evidence for inhibition by brain serotonin of mouse killing behavior in rats. Nature 233:272–273, 1971

Elphick M, Yang JD, Cowen PJ: Effects of carbamazepine on dopamine- and serotonin-mediated neuroendocrine responses. Arch Gen Psychiatry 47:135–140, 1990

Goldberg SC, Schulz SC, Schulz PM, et al: Borderline and schizotypal personality disorders treated with low-dose thiothixene versus placebo. Arch Gen Psychiatry 43:680–686, 1986

Goodman WK, Price LH, Delgado PL, et al: Specificity of serotonin reuptake inhibitors in the treatment of obsessive-compulsive disorder: comparison of fluvoxamine and desipramine. Arch Gen Psychiatry 47:577–585, 1990

Gross-Isseroff R, Dillon KA, Fieldust SJ, et al: Autoradiographic analysis of alpha1-noradrenergic receptors in the human brain postmortem: effect of suicide. Arch Gen Psychiatry 47:1049–1053, 1990

Herman BH, Hammock MK, Arthur-Smith BS, et al: Naltrexone decreases self-injurious behavior. Ann Neurol 22:550–552, 1987

Higley JD, Mehlman PT, Taub DM, et al: Cerebrospinal fluid monoamine and adrenal correlates of aggression in free-ranging rhesus monkeys. Arch Gen Psychiatry 49:436–441, 1992

Hollander E, DeCaria CM, Gully R, et al: Effects of chronic fluoxetine treatment on behavioral and neuroendocrine responses to metachlorophenylpiperazine in obsessive-compulsive disorder. Psychiatry Res 36:1–17, 1991a

Hollander E, DeCaria CM, Nitescu A, et al: Noradrenergic function in obsessive-compulsive disorder: behavioral and neuroendocrine responses to clonidine and comparison to healthy controls. Psychiatry Res 37:161–177, 1991b

Hollander E, DeCaria CM, Nitescu A, et al: Serotonergic function in obsessive-compulsive disorder: behavioral and neuroendocrine responses to oral m-chlorophenylpiperazine and fenfluramine in patients and healthy volunteers. Arch Gen Psychiatry 49:21–28, 1992a

Hollander E, Frenkel M, DeCaria CM, et al: Treatment of pathological gambling with clomipramine (letter). Am J Psychiatry 149:710–711, 1992b

Hollander E, Stein DJ, DeCaria CM, et al: Serotonergic sensitivity in borderline personality disorder: preliminary findings. Am J Psychiatry 151:277–280, 1994

Kafantaris V, Campbell M, Padron-Gayol MV, et al: Carbamazepine in hospitalized aggressive conduct disorder children: an open pilot study. Psychopharmacol Bull 28:193–199, 1992

Kantak KM, Hegstrand LR, Eichelman BR: Facilitation of shock induced fighting following intraventricular 5,7-dihydroxytryptamine and 6-hydroxydopa. Psychopharmacology (Berl) 74:157–160, 1981

Kavoussi RJ, Liu J, Coccaro EF: Sertraline in the treatment of impulsive aggression in personality disordered patients. J Clin Psychiatry 55:137–141, 1994

Kruesi MJ: Cruelty to animals and CSF 5-HIAA. Psychiatry Res 28: 115–116, 1989

Kruesi MJ, Rapoport JL, Hamburger S, et al: Cerebrospinal fluid monoamine metabolites, aggression, and impulsivity in disruptive behavior disorders of children and adolescents. Arch Gen Psychiatry 47:419–426, 1990

Lee MA, Cameron OG, Gurguis GN, et al: Alpha$_2$-adrenoreceptor status in obsessive-compulsive disorder. Biol Psychiatry 27:1083–1093, 1990

Lesch KP, Hoh A, Disselkamp-Tietze J, et al: 5-Hydroxytryptamine$_{1A}$ receptor responsivity in obsessive-compulsive disorder: comparison of patients and controls. Arch Gen Psychiatry 48:540–547, 1991

Links PS, Steiner M, Boiago I, et al: Lithium therapy for borderline patients: findings. Journal of Personality Disorders 4:173–181, 1990

Linnoila M, Virkkunen M, Scheinin M, et al: Low cerebrospinal fluid 5-hydroxyindoleacetic acid concentration differentiates impulsive from nonimpulsive violent behavior. Life Sci 33:2609–2614, 1983

Lucey JV, Butcher G, Clare AW, et al: Buspirone induced prolactin responses in obsessive-compulsive disorder (OCD): is OCD a 5-HT$_2$ receptor disorder? Int Clin Psychopharmacol 7:45–49, 1992a

Lucey JV, O'Keane V, Butcher G, et al: Cortisol and prolactin responses to d-fenfluramine in non-depressed patients with obsessive-compulsive disorder: a comparison with depressed and healthy controls. Br J Psychiatry 161:517–521, 1992b

Mancini C, Brown GM: Urinary catecholamines and cortisol in parasuicide. Psychiatry Res 43:31–42, 1992

Mann JJ, Stanley M, McBride PA, et al: Increased serotonin$_2$ and beta-adrenergic receptor binding in frontal cortices of suicide victims. Arch Gen Psychiatry 43:954–959, 1986

Marazziti D, Hollander E, Lensi P, et al: Peripheral markers of serotonin and dopamine function in obsessive-compulsive disorder. Psychiatry Res 42:41–51, 1992

Mattes JA: Propranolol for adults with temper outbursts and residual attention-deficit disorder. J Clin Psychopharmacol 6:299–302, 1986

Mattes JA: Valproic acid for nonaffective aggression in the mentally retarded. J Nerv Ment Dis 180:601–602, 1992

McBride PA, DeMeo MD, Sweeney JA, et al: Neuroendocrine and behavioral responses to challenge with the indirect serotonin agonist dl-fenfluramine in adults with obsessive-compulsive disorder. Biol Psychiatry 31:19–34, 1992

McElroy SL, Hudson JI Jr, Pope HG Jr, et al: The DSM-III-R Impulse control disorders not elsewhere classified: clinical characteristics and relationship to other psychiatric disorders. Am J Psychiatry 149:318–327, 1992

Mehlman PT, Higley JD, Faucher I, et al: Low CSF 5-HIAA concentrations and severe aggression and impaired impulse control in nonhuman primates. Am J Psychiatry 151:1485–1491, 1994

Mizuno T, Yugari Y: Self-mutilation in Lesch-Nyhan syndrome. Lancet 1:761, 1974

Montgomery SA, Montgomery D: Pharmacological prevention of suicidal behavior. J Affect Disord 4:219–298, 1982

Moss HB, Yao JK, Panzak GL: Serotonergic responsivity and behavioral dimensions in antisocial personality disorder with substance abuse. Biol Psychiatry 28:325–338, 1990

Nielsen DA, Goldman D, Virkkunen M, et al: Suicidality and 5-hydroxyindoleacetic acid concentration associated with a tryptophan hydroxylase polymorphism. Arch Gen Psychiatry 51:34–38, 1994

Norden MJ: Fluoxetine in borderline personality disorder. Prog Neuropsychopharmacol Biol Psychiatry 13:885–893, 1989

Pandey SC, Kim SW, Davis JM, et al: Platelet serotonin2 receptors in obsessive-compulsive disorder. Biol Psychiatry 33:367–372, 1993

Parsons B, Quitkin FM, McGrath PJ, et al: Phenelzine, imipramine, and placebo in borderline patients meeting criteria for atypical depression. Psychopharmacol Bull 25:524–534, 1989

Patel H, Bruza D, Yeragani VK: Treatment of self-abusive behavior with trazodone (letter). Can J Psychiatry 33:331–332, 1988

Pato MT, Pigott TA, Hill JL, et al: Controlled comparison of buspirone and clomipramine in obsessive-compulsive disorder. Am J Psychiatry 148:127–129, 1991

Pigott TA, Pato MT, Bernstein SE, et al: Controlled comparisons of clomipramine and fluoxetine in the treatment of obsessive-compulsive disorder: behavioral and biological results. Arch Gen Psychiatry 47:926–932, 1990

Pigott TA, Zohar J, Hill JL, et al: Metergoline blocks the behavioral and neuroendocrine effects of orally administered m-chlorophenylpiperazine in patients with obsessive-compulsive disorder. Biol Psychiatry 29:418–426, 1991

Pollard CA, Ibe IO, Krojanker DN, et al: Clomipramine treatment of trichotillomania: a follow-up report on four cases. J Clin Psychiatry 52:128–130, 1991

Pratt JA, Jenner P, Johnson AL, et al: Anticonvulsant drugs alter plasma tryptophan concentrations in epileptic patients: implications for antiepileptic action and mental function. J Neurol Neurosurg Psychiatry 47:1131-1133, 1984

Ratey JJ, Sovner R, Parks A, et al: Buspirone treatment of aggression and anxiety in mentally retarded patients: a multiple baseline, placebo lead-in study. J Clin Psychiatry 52:159-161, 1991

Ratey JJ, Sorgi P, O'Driscoll GA, et al: Nadolol to treat aggression and psychiatric symptomatology in chronic psychiatric inpatients: a double-blind, placebo-controlled study. J Clin Psychiatry 53:41-46, 1992

Rifkin A, Quitkin F, Carrillo C, et al: Lithium carbonate in emotionally unstable character disorder. Arch Gen Psychiatry 27:519-523, 1972

Roy A, Adinoff B, Roehrich L, et al: Pathological gambling: a psychobiological study. Arch Gen Psychiatry 45:369-373, 1988

Roy A, DeJong J, Linnoila M: Extroversion in pathologic gamblers: correlates with indexes of noradrenergic function. Arch Gen Psychiatry 46:679-681, 1989

Sheard MH, Marini JL, Bridges CI, et al: The effect of lithium on impulsive aggressive behavior in man. Am J Psychiatry 133:1409-1413, 1976

Soloff PH, George A, Nathan RS, et al: Paradoxical effects of amitriptyline in borderline patients. Am J Psychiatry 143:1603-1605, 1986

Soloff PH, George A, Nathan RS, et al: Amitriptyline versus haloperidol in borderlines: final outcomes and predictors of response. J Clin Psychopharmacol 9:238-246, 1989

Sorgi PJ, Ratey JJ, Polakoff S: Beta-adrenergic blockers for the control of aggressive behaviors in patients with chronic schizophrenia. Am J Psychiatry 143:775-776, 1986

Stanley M, Viggilio J, Gershon S: Tritiated imipramine binding sites are decreased in the frontal cortex of suicides. Science 216:1337-1339, 1982

Stein DJ, Hollander E, Anthony DT, et al: Serotonergic medications for sexual obsessions, sexual addictions, and paraphilias. J Clin Psychiatry 53:267-271, 1992

Swedo SE, Leonard HL, Rappoport JL, et al: A double-blind comparison of clomipramine and desipramine in the treatment of trichotillomania. N Engl J Med 321:497-501, 1989

Teicher MH, Glod CA, Aaronson ST, et al: Open assessment of the safety and efficacy of thioridazine in the treatment of patients with borderline personality disorder. Psychopharmacol Bull 25:535-549, 1989

Träskman-Bendz L, Alling C, Oreland L, et al: Prediction of suicidal behavior from biologic tests. J Clin Psychopharmacol 12(suppl):21-26, 1992

Tupin J, Smith D, Clanon T, et al: The long-term use of lithium in aggressive prisoners. Compr Psychiatry 14:311–317, 1973

van Praag HM: (Auto)aggression and CSF 5-HIAA in depression and schizophrenia. Psychopharmacol Bull 22:669–673, 1986

Virkkunen M, Nuutila A, Goodwin FK, et al: Cerebrospinal fluid monoamine metabolite levels in male arsonists. Arch Gen Psychiatry 44:241–247, 1987

Virkkunen M, DeJong J, Bartko J, et al: Psychobiological concomitants of history of suicide attempts among violent offenders and impulsive fire setters. Arch Gen Psychiatry 46:604–606, 1989

Vitiello B, Shimon H, Behar D, et al: Platelet imipramine binding and serotonin uptake in obsessive-compulsive patients. Acta Psychiatr Scand 84:29–32, 1991

Wender PH, Reimherr FW: Bupropion treatment of attention-deficit hyperactivity disorder in adults. Am J Psychiatry 147:1018–1020, 1990

Wender PH, Reimherr FW, Wood DR: Attention-deficit disorder ("minimal brain dysfunction") in adults: a replication study of diagnosis and drug treatment. Arch Gen Psychiatry 38:449–456, 1981

Winchel RM, Stanley M: Self-injurious behavior: a review of the behavior and biology of self-mutilation. Am J Psychiatry 148:306–317, 1991

Yudofsky SC, Williams D, Gorman J: Propranolol in the treatment of rage and violent behavior in patients with chronic brain syndromes. Am J Psychiatry 138:218–220, 1981

# 6

## Psychobiology and Psychopharmacology of Compulsive Spectrum Disorders

Eric Hollander, M.D.
Lisa J. Cohen, Ph.D.

I n recent years there has been increased interest in the concept
of an obsessive-compulsive spectrum of disorders (Hollander
1993b), a group of disorders that show significant overlap in clinical symptoms, associated features (e.g., age of onset, comorbidity,
course of illness), family history, and possibly preferential response
to serotonin reuptake inhibitors and specific forms of behavior
therapy. One important dimension within this spectrum is the
compulsive-impulsive dimension (Figure 6–1).

Supported in part by Research Scientist Development Award MH-00750 to Dr.
Hollander from the National Institute of Mental Health, Bethesda, Maryland.

The compulsive endpoint in this dimension involves a heightened estimation of harm and risk avoidance. The impulsive endpoint in this dimension involves a decreased sense of the harmful consequences of one's behavior along with elevated risk-seeking behavior. Biological models of the compulsive spectrum are supported by evidence from studies of serotonin function, brain imaging, neurological soft signs, and neuropsychological function. Complementary findings on impulsive disorders further support a dimensional approach to compulsivity and impulsivity.

Compulsive disorders are characterized phenomenologically by an increased sense of harm avoidance, risk aversiveness, and anticipatory anxiety. These disorders may include obsessive-compulsive disorder (OCD), body dysmorphic disorder, anorexia nervosa, depersonalization disorder, hypochondriasis, and Tourette's disorder. In these illnesses, ritualistic behaviors are often undertaken

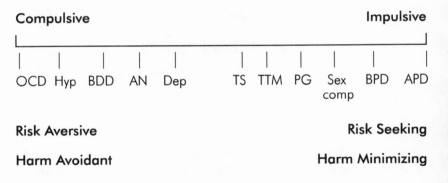

**Figure 6–1.** Impulsive-compulsive spectrum characterized by dimensions of risk-aversive/risk-seeking and harm-avoidant/harm-minimizing behaviors. Disorders on the compulsive end of the spectrum include obsessive-compulsive disorder (OCD), hypochondriasis (Hyp), body dysmorphic disorder (BDD), anorexia nervosa (AN), and depersonalization (Dep). Mixed compulsive and impulsive disorders include Tourette's disorder (Tourette's syndrome [TS]), trichotillomania (TTM), pathological gambling (PG), and sexual compulsions (Sex comp). Disorders on the impulsive end of the spectrum include borderline personality disorder (BPD) and antisocial personality disorder (APD). *Source.* Adapted from Hollander 1993a.

in an attempt to reduce anxiety and magically decrease the sense of harm or risk (Figure 6–2).

In contrast, impulsive disorders are characterized by risk-seeking behavior, a defect in harm avoidance, and little anticipatory anxiety. These disorders may include personality disorders characterized by impulsive aggression, such as Cluster B personality disorders (i.e., borderline, antisocial, histrionic, narcissistic); disorders of impulse control (e.g., intermittent explosive disorder, pyromania, kleptomania, pathological gambling, and trichotillomania); and paraphilias and sexual acting-out behaviors (Figure 6–2). These disorders are characterized by pleasure-producing behaviors, although the consequences of such behavior may be painful.

Nevertheless, a hallmark of both classes of disorders is the inability to delay or inhibit repetitive behaviors. This is also a key feature of obsessive-compulsive spectrum disorders in general (Figure 6–2). In compulsive disorders, such behaviors have a driven quality and function mainly to reduce anxiety or tension. Impulsive behaviors are usually experienced as pleasurable. However, the common feature involves the repetitive nature of the behavior and the impairment in inhibition.

Nevertheless, this distinction is not always so clear-cut. Some disorders may have both impulsive and compulsive features or lie between these two poles. Thus, patients with trichotillomania and pathological gambling may have both compulsive and impulsive features, in that their behavior may have a driven, tension-reducing quality as well as pleasurable characteristics (Figure 6–1).

# Psychobiology of Compulsive Disorders

## Neurotransmitter Function

Considerable evidence implicates serotonergic dysfunction in the neurobiology of compulsive disorders. Many studies suggest increased serotonergic tone in compulsive disorder, in contrast to decreased serotonergic tone found in impulsive disorders.

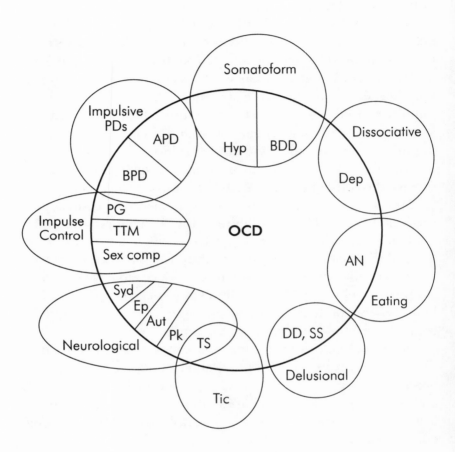

**Figure 6–2.** Overlap between obsessive-compulsive disorder (OCD) and somatoform, dissociative, eating, delusional, tic, neurological, impulse-control, and impulsive personality disorders. Abbreviations (*clockwise from top*): Hyp = hypochondriasis; BDD = body dysmorphic disorder; Dep = depersonalization; AN = anorexia nervosa; DD,SS = delusional disorder, somatic subtype; TS = Tourette's syndrome (Tourette's disorder); Pk = Parkinson's disease; Aut = autism; Ep = epilepsy; Syd = Sydenham's chorea; Sex comp = sexual compulsions; TTM = trichotillomania; PG = pathological gambling; PDs = personality disorders; BPD = borderline personality disorder; APD = antisocial personality disorder.   *Source.* Adapted from Hollander 1993a.

Serotonergic function may be measured by cerebrospinal fluid (CSF) metabolites of serotonin (5-hydroxytryptamine; 5-HT), such as 5-hydroxyindoleacetic acid (5-HIAA); by behavioral and neuroendocrine responses to serotonergic probes (m-chlorophenylpiperazine [m-CPP] and others); and by treatment outcome to serotonin reuptake inhibitors (i.e., fluoxetine, clomipramine, fluvoxamine, and others). Compulsive disorders such as OCD (Insel et al. 1985; Thorén et al. 1980) and anorexia nervosa (Kaye et al. 1991) are correlated with increased concentrations of 5-HIAA overall, or in subgroups of patients responsive to serotonin reuptake inhibitors. On the other hand, patients with impulsive aggressive (Linnoila et al. 1983) and violent suicidal (Åsberg et al. 1976) behavior have decreased CSF 5-HIAA concentrations. Patients who had completed violent suicide were found to have a decreased number of serotonin receptors in frontal cortex (Arora and Meltzer 1989).

In response to serotonin agonists such as m-CPP, patients with compulsive disorders such as OCD (Hollander et al. 1992c; Zohar et al. 1987), eating disorders (Buttinger et al. 1990), and Tourette's disorder (E. Hollander, C. M. DeCaria, M. Hwang, et al., unpublished observations, 1992) show increased dysphoria and increased obsessional thoughts and compulsive urges. A blunted prolactin response to m-CPP has also been demonstrated in a subgroup of OCD patients (Hollander et al. 1992c), which suggests dysregulation of the serotonergic system. On the other hand, impulsive personality disorder patients for the most part do not show a dysphoric response, but rather often have increased ratings of "high" in response to m-CPP (Hollander et al. 1994). Neuroendocrine blunting in response to serotonin agonists (Coccaro et al. 1989) has also been demonstrated in impulsive patients.

In response to serotonin reuptake inhibitors, patients with compulsive disorders such as OCD, anorexia nervosa, hypochondriasis, body dysmorphic disorder, and depersonalization disorder show clear-cut and often dramatic improvement with chronic treatment. Because serotonin reuptake inhibitors function to stimulate serotonergic activity, symptoms may initially worsen following acute administration with high doses (Hollander et al. 1992b).

Chronic treatment with these agents, however, may work to desensitize or downregulate serotonin receptors over time (Hollander et al. 1991b; Zohar et al. 1988). Disorders with mixed impulsive and compulsive features, such as trichotillomania, show early improvement after administration of serotonin reuptake inhibitors (Swedo et al. 1989), although this effect has also been reported to wear off with time (Pollard et al. 1991). Open pilot work in impulsive personality disorders shows some improvement early on after administration of serotonin reuptake inhibitors (Coccaro et al. 1990), but this effect may also wear off with time, and long-term follow-up studies are needed. One might postulate that acute administration of serotonin reuptake inhibitors might worsen compulsive but improve impulsive disorders, whereas chronic administration of these agents might improve compulsive but ultimately worsen impulsive disorders.

Although the evidence of serotonergic dysregulation in compulsive disorders is substantial, heterogeneity on such dysfunction is suggested by the finding that only 60% of patients have a good response to a single trial of a serotonin reuptake inhibitor. In OCD patients, lack of treatment response to either clomipramine ($n = 6$) or fluoxetine ($n = 10$) was associated with increased behavioral exacerbation and severe prolactin blunting following challenge with m-CPP. This suggests that patients with very severe serotonergic system abnormalities may be less responsive to attempts at normalization with serotonin reuptake inhibitors (Hollander et al. 1993b).

Dopaminergic mechanisms may also be involved in compulsive disorders, particularly those with simple motor symptoms, such as Tourette's disorder (Shapiro and Shapiro 1988) or trichotillomania (Stein and Hollander 1992), or those with psychotic features, such as body dysmorphic disorder or delusional OCD (Hollander et al. 1989).

## Neuroanatomic Studies

Abnormalities in brain structure and function have been demonstrated in imaging studies with positron-emission tomography

(PET), single-photon emission computed tomography (SPECT), computed tomography (CT), and electroencephalography. Hyperfrontality, in particular, has been consistently documented in compulsive disorders such as OCD (Insel 1992). In OCD patients, there is evidence of increased metabolic activity (Baxter et al. 1987) and blood flow (Rubin et al. 1992) to the frontal lobes. Further, the hyperfrontality appears related to severity of compulsions (Rubin et al. 1992; Swedo et al. 1992) and is increased by behavioral (Zohar et al. 1989) and acute serotonergic pharmacological (Hollander et al. 1991c) challenges, which increase compulsive symptoms. Increased frontal activity on SPECT has also been demonstrated in case reports of depersonalization disorder (Hollander et al. 1992a) and body dysmorphic disorder (L. J. Cohen, E. Hollander, C. M. DeCaria, et al., unpublished observations, 1993).

The hyperfrontality demonstrated in OCD has been shown to be decreased (normalized) following chronic serotonin reuptake inhibitor treatment, and this normalization is associated with decreased harm avoidance (Hoehn-Saric et al. 1991). Neurosurgical procedures such as anterior capsulotomy and cingulotomy decrease frontal lobe input to the limbic system and are effective in patients with severely refractory OCD (Jenike et al. 1991). Of interest, hypofrontality from prefrontal lobotomies may, in some cases, even result in a lack of anticipatory anxiety and harm avoidance, and the development of psychopathic features (Valenstein 1986).

Notably, impulsive patients, such as patients with borderline personality disorder, were shown in one study to have decreased frontal glucose metabolic rates, and those with greater aggression had lower frontal activity (Goyer et al. 1991).

In summary, compulsivity, defined by an increased sense of harm and risk, may be mediated by hyperfrontality and hyperserotonergic function. In contrast, impulsivity, defined by a defect in the ability to sense and avoid harm, may be mediated by hypofrontality and hyposerotonergic function.

Abnormal function in the basal ganglia has also been implicated in compulsive disorders. In OCD patients, elevated caudate activity on PET was normalized following either behavior therapy or treatment with fluoxetine (Baxter et al. 1992). Abnormal activity in the putamen was demonstrated on PET in Tourette's disorder patients. These findings suggest that anterior basal ganglia impairment, with greater input from frontal cortex, may be associated with cognitive symptoms (obsessions and complex compulsions), whereas more ventral impairment leads to simple motor symptoms (tics or simple tapping compulsions).

## Neuropsychiatric Investigations

Investigations of neurological soft signs and neuropsychological function have documented a range of neuropsychiatric impairments in the compulsive disorders spectrum.

Neurological soft signs are nonlocalizing signs of deviant performance on a motor or sensory test when no other sign of a neurological lesion is present (Tupper 1987). Abnormalities include disorders of coordination, involuntary movements, and sensory signs. Early studies demonstrated increased soft signs in emotionally unstable character disorder (Quitkin et al. 1976).

We found that a subgroup of OCD patients have increased neurological soft signs (Hollander et al. 1990b); these patients may have more severe illness (Hollander et al. 1990b), increased ventricular size on CT (Stein et al. 1993a), greater familial transmission of soft signs (Aronowitz et al. 1992), and a worse treatment outcome with serotonin reuptake inhibitors (Hollander et al. 1993b). Follow-up studies of children with increased neurological soft signs have demonstrated the development of adult OCD, affective disorders, and anxiety disorders (Hollander et al. 1991a).

We also studied the relationship between soft signs and neurological functions in patients with impulsive personality disorders (Stein et al. 1993b). Although patients had more left-sided soft signs than did control subjects, those with a history of aggression had more right-sided soft signs than did those without a history of aggression. Furthermore, right-sided soft signs were predictive of measures of executive dysfunction.

The most consistent neuropsychological finding in OCD involves impairment in visuospatial functions, including visual-memory and visual-constructional ability (Aronowitz et al. 1994; Boone et al. 1991; Christensen et al. 1992; Head et al. 1989; Zielinski et al. 1991; L. J. Cohen, E. Hollander, C. M. DeCaria, et al., unpublished observations, 1995). Although there is some suggestion of impaired executive function (i.e., ability to form, maintain, and switch cognitive sets) in OCD, findings are inconclusive and measures often include visuospatial components (Behar et al. 1984; Boone et al. 1991; Christensen et al. 1992; Flor-Henry et al. 1979; Head et al. 1989; Martinot et al. 1990; Zielinski et al. 1991). Impairment in immediate auditory recall (Wechsler Adult Intelligence Scale—Revised (WAIS-R) Digit Span) has been demonstrated in some studies (Behar et al. 1984; Martinot et al. 1990) but not others (Boone et al. 1991; Hollander et al. 1990b), and visual but not verbal memory deficits have been reported (Zielinski et al. 1991). Finally, attentional problems have been documented in some but not all OCD patients (Behar et al. 1984; Martinot et al. 1990; Zielinski et al. 1991).

Impaired executive function would be consistent with the hyperfrontality found in imaging studies. However, most tests of executive dysfunction are sensitive to frontal hypoactivity, and little is known about the functional correlates of elevated frontal activity. The deficits in visual-constructional ability may implicate motor function, which would be consistent with basal ganglia abnormalities.

Broad visuospatial deficits, however, also suggest right-hemisphere abnormalities, which have not been documented on imaging studies. Nonetheless, the notion of right-hemisphere dysfunction is consistent with findings of increased left-hemibody soft signs in OCD (Hollander et al. 1991d). Furthermore, the pattern of impaired visuospatial functions relative to language functions complements the pattern of lateralization found in some impulsive disorders, in which language skills are impaired relative to visuospatial skills (Moffitt and Henry 1991). This is also consistent with the association between right-sided soft signs and history of aggression found in impulsive personality disorder patients (Stein et al. 1993b).

There are fewer data on neuropsychological function in other compulsive disorders. Social phobic patients, who show increased risk aversion regarding interpersonal evaluation, have also demonstrated executive and visuospatial dysfunction (L. J. Cohen, E. Hollander, C. M. DeCaria, et al., unpublished observations, 1995). Patients with Tourette's disorder performed more than one standard deviation below standardized means only on tests of motor function (Bornstein and Yang 1991), a finding that is consistent with basal ganglia impairment.

In summary, studies of neurological soft signs and neuropsychological function have documented neuropsychiatric impairment in a number of compulsive as well as impulsive disorders. These findings may further elucidate the biological underpinnings of the compulsive-impulsive spectrum.

## Treatment Considerations

Drug treatment studies may suggest pharmacological dissection between impulsivity and compulsivity. Compulsive style disorders such as OCD (The Clomipramine Collaborative Study Group 1991), body dysmorphic disorder (Hollander 1993b; Hollander et al. 1989, 1993a; Phillips et al. 1993), hypochondriasis (Fallon et al. 1993), depersonalization disorder (Hollander et al. 1990a), and anorexia nervosa (Kaye et al. 1991) may respond preferentially to serotonin reuptake inhibitors. It remains to be seen whether impulsive-style disorders, such as pathological gambling (Hollander et al. 1992d) and sexual compulsions and paraphilias (Stein et al. 1992), and impulsive-style personality disorders (Coccaro et al. 1990) have an equally preferential responsivity to this treatment approach. For example, true sexual obsessions, a typical subtype of OCD, are highly responsive to serotonin reuptake inhibitor treatment, whereas paraphilias and sexual impulsions have a less robust and shorter response to this treatment (Stein et al. 1992). Trichotillomania, which has both compulsive and impulsive qualities, may have an intermediate response, with good initial response to (Swedo et al. 1989) but unclear long-term outcome with this treatment (Pollard et al. 1991; Stein and Hollander 1992).

Despite advances in the treatment of compulsive disorders, most patients attain only partial relief from their symptoms. In addition, about 40% of OCD patients remain refractory to a single trial of a standard serotonin reuptake inhibitor.

Pharmacological factors in treatment resistance include insufficient dosage (less than 250 mg clomipramine equivalents), slow onset of response (12 weeks are often needed) (The Clomipramine Collaborative Study Group 1991), inadequate duration of treatment (at least 12 months are often necessary for initial treatment length), and symptom relapse after discontinuation. Treatment resistance may also result from inadequate treatment of comorbid Axis II conditions, such as Cluster A (odd) or B (impulsive) personality disorders, social phobia, or tics or neurological illness. Obsessions of delusional severity also may impede treatment efficacy.

An algorithm for the pharmacological approach to compulsive patients is presented in Figure 6–3. The first-line strategy is a trial of clomipramine or a selective serotonin reuptake inhibitor (SSRI) (fluvoxamine, fluoxetine, sertraline, paroxetine). Augmentation strategies for patients with incomplete response to clomipramine or a single SSRI include adding one of a variety of agents to the SSRI or combining clomipramine with another serotonin reuptake inhibitor. Buspirone (30–60 mg/day) or clonazepam (1–8 mg/day) for anxious OCD patients, fenfluramine (20–60 mg/day) or desipramine (10–30 mg/day) for depressed OCD patients, and carbamazepine (200–1,800 mg/day) or lithium for bipolar OCD patients have all been reported to be helpful augmentation strategies in some patients with refractory OCD (Hollander and Cohen 1994). When an SSRI, such as fluoxetine, fluvoxamine, sertraline, or paroxetine, is being added to clomipramine, it is important to follow the combined clomipramine and desmethylclomipramine blood levels, which should not exceed a combined level of 1,000 ng/mL to avoid an increased risk of seizures. In addition, intensive behavior therapy is a highly effective augmentation strategy for refractory OCD (Hollander and Cohen 1994).

Behavior therapy has been shown to have considerable efficacy in the treatment of compulsive disorders (Josephson and Brondolo 1993; Neziroglu and Yaryura-Tobias 1993). The technique of

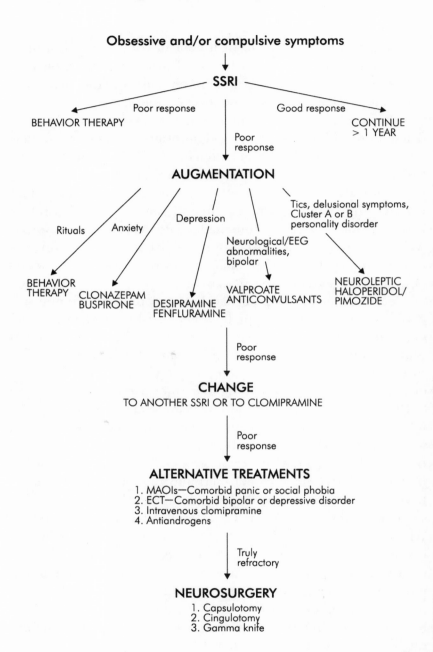

**Figure 6–3.**   Treatment of compulsive disorders. SSRI = selective serotonin reuptake inhibitor; EEG = electroencephalogram; MAOI = monoamine oxidase inhibitor; ECT = electroconvulsive therapy.

exposure and response prevention (ERP) was first shown to be effective with OCD patients (Foa and Steketee 1989). This technique involves graduated exposure to the feared stimulus with simultaneous prevention of ritualistic behaviors designed to reduce anxiety. The patient thus becomes desensitized to the anxiety-provoking stimulus and no longer relies on the compulsions to regulate anxiety. ERP combined with cognitive therapy to decrease distortions in self-perceptions has also been found to be effective in a series of patients with body dysmorphic disorder (Neziroglu and Yaryura-Tobias 1993). In trichotillomania, behavior therapy techniques aim to increase the patient's awareness of the symptomatic behavior in order to make it accessible to conscious control. Habit reversal, which involves identification of the behavioral antecedents and then substitution with a less problematic behavior (e.g., fist clenching), has been reported to be effective with trichotillomanic patients (Azrin et al. 1980). The different focus of the two techniques (increased awareness vs. decreased anticipatory anxiety) may reflect the impulsive features of trichotillomania.

# Clinical Profile and Case Examples

In this section we discuss examples of treatment approaches to particularly difficult cases of patients with specific compulsive disorders.

## Obsessive-Compulsive Disorder

Classified in DSM-IV (American Psychiatric Association 1994) as an anxiety disorder, OCD is characterized by obsessions (i.e., intrusive, senseless, and repetitive thoughts, typically anxiety provoking) and/or compulsions (i.e., repetitive, stereotyped rituals, typically anxiety reducing). OCD has an early onset, a chronic course, and a preferential response to serotonin reuptake inhibitors and ERP, a specific form of behavior therapy that was discussed in the preceding section (Foa and Steketee 1989).

■ Case 1: "Fear of 13"—Refractory OCD

A 34-year-old woman presented with obsessions of causing future harm by touching, arranging, or moving objects "on the number 13." Associated numbering, repeating, and tapping compulsions were intended to undo any action performed "on 13." Subsequent avoidance of feared behaviors precluded many aspects of daily functioning and left this patient essentially housebound. A secondary obsession concerned being too pretty or showy and eliciting rageful reactions from her mother. This secondary obsession resulted in avoidance of jewelry and other bodily adornments. Comorbid disorders included depression and body dysmorphic disorder (preoccupation with her father's ideal of small breasts and large hips). Thirteen years of psychoanalytic psychotherapy increased autonomous functioning but did not affect OCD symptomatology. After 1 year of fluoxetine 20 mg/day, her OCD symptoms, as measured by the Yale-Brown Obsessive Compulsive Scale (Goodman et al. 1989a, 1989b), were unchanged. A gradual increase to fluoxetine 80 mg/day resulted in minimal improvement in OCD severity. Fluoxetine 40 mg/day was augmented with clomipramine 100 mg/day, clonazepam 3 mg/day, and weekly supportive/behavior therapy. Combined clomipramine/desmethylclomipramine levels were 600 ng/mL. Within 1 month the patient reported much improvement in OCD symptom frequency, severity, and duration. These gains held for more than 6 months of follow-up.

## Body Dysmorphic Disorder

Body dysmorphic disorder, which is characterized by an excessive concern with perceived defects in bodily appearance, is classified in DSM-IV as a somatoform disorder. Areas of concern focus primarily on the face and head but also include hands, feet, the torso, and sexual body parts. Related behaviors included mirror checking, ritualized grooming behaviors, repeated requests for reassurance, and even requesting and undergoing multiple cosmetic surgeries. Avoidance of social and occupational situations for fear of exacerbating or exposing perceived defects is also common. Body dysmorphic disorder ideation may vary along a continuum of insight. In DSM-IV, delusional body dysmorphic disorder ideation earns a comorbid diagnosis of delusional disorder, somatic type. Although, to date, there are no controlled treatment studies, preliminary investigations point to a preferential response to serotonin reuptake inhibitors (Hollander et al. 1989, 1993a; Phillips et al. 1993). In delusional patients, neuroleptic augmentation may be useful (Cohen et al. 1994; Hollander et al. 1989).

■ Case 2: "The Fatty Buttocks"—Body Dysmorphic Disorder

A 26-year-old man first experienced body dysmorphic disorder symptoms in childhood but had an acute exacerbation in late adolescence. Initial concerns about the width of his nose led to excessive mirror checking and social withdrawal. A rhinoplasty temporarily alleviated his distress, although new concerns developed, specifically about asymmetry in his testicles and fatty deposits on his buttocks. Along with intensified mirror checking, social withdrawal, and secondary depression, these symptoms led to other surgical procedures (surgery to enhance testicular symmetry and liposuction on buttocks). Comorbid OCD included obsessions about orderliness, symmetry, and contamination, as well as checking and arranging compulsions. His mother and grandmother also had OCD. Desipramine 250 mg/day for 2 months failed to improve either the body dysmorphic disorder or depression. A 4-month trial of nortriptyline 125 mg/day and trifluoperazine 4 mg/day decreased the severity of the depression but did not change the body dysmorphic disorder symptoms. The patient remained housebound. Clomipramine 150 mg/day resulted in decreased depression and partial improvement in the body dysmorphic disorder. However, weight gain and sedation presented troublesome side effects. Fluvoxamine 300 mg/day led to marked improvement in both the body dysmorphic disorder and the depressive symptoms and was well tolerated. The patient was able to obtain employment and socialize. These gains remained after 4 years.

## Trichotillomania

Trichotillomania, classified in DSM-IV as an impulse-control disorder, is characterized by the repeated urge to pull out one's hair. There is debate over this classification, because trichotillomania presents compulsive as well as impulsive features (Hollander 1993b; Swedo 1993b). Compulsive features are suggested by similarities between trichotillomania and OCD in phenomenology and neurobiology. These similarities include the inability to inhibit repetitive, ego-dystonic behavior (Hollander 1993b; Swedo 1993b), high comorbidity between the two disorders (Christenson et al. 1991; Cohen et al. 1995), and possible serotonergic mediation (Swedo et al. 1989; Thorén et al. 1980).

Impulsive features in patients with trichotillomania include evidence of pleasurable feelings following symptomatic behavior (Swedo and Leonard 1992), a high rate of comorbid personality disorders (Swedo 1993a), and patterns of serotonergic function consistent with impulsive disorders, such as indication of early treatment response to serotonin reuptake inhibitors with long-term relapse (Pollard et al. 1991), and mood elevation in response to serotonergic probes (Stein et al., in press).

■ Case 3: "Sometimes I feel like pulling my hair out"—Trichotillomania

A 26-year-old woman, using only her left hand, pulled several hundred hairs daily from her scalp (crown, front, sides) and pubic area. Bald spots were disguised with brown hair spray and hair extensions. The patient reported no associated ideation except a trancelike feeling of "paralysis." Although pulling increased when the patient felt stressed or depressed, most pulling occurred in relaxed conditions. Onset was at age 8 years, when she began pulling hairs in increasing sets of 3's. Comorbid disorders included depression, panic disorder with agoraphobia, and borderline personality disorder. Onset of OCD (blasphemous thoughts of Jesus), now in remission, preceded onset of the trichotillomania. A 1-year trial of fluoxetine 60 mg/day decreased panic attacks but increased impulsivity, irritability, muscle spasms, and suicidal ideation. A 2-year trial of clomipramine 250 mg/day resulted in weight gain of 55 pounds. Augmentation with lithium 300 mg/day decreased the trichotillomanic symptoms and resolved the weight gain but produced migraine aura. Two years of clonazepam 1 mg/day, propranolol 20 mg/day, and lorazepam 1 mg prn decreased anxiety but not the trichotillomanic symptoms. Four months after addition of weekly supportive/behavior therapy to this last regimen, the trichotillomanic symptoms decreased to about 40 hairs pulled per day, allowing the patient to remove her hair extensions.

## Depersonalization

Depersonalization disorder, classified in DSM-IV as a dissociative disorder, is characterized by a subjective sense of unreality or disconnection from one's own body, mentation, feelings, or action. Depersonalized experiences are often associated with depression, anxiety, severe stress, or trauma (Simeon and Hollander 1993). Depersonalization disorder has been conceptualized as an obsessive-compulsive–related disorder falling on the compulsive end of the impulsive-compulsive spectrum (Figure 6–1). Although depersonalization is not characterized by repetitive behaviors per se, obsessive-compulsive features include preoccupation with and repetitive experiences of altered sensory perceptions and feelings of detachment (cf. Skodol and Oldham, Chapter 1, this volume). Serotonergic involvement is suggested by reports of symptom precipitation following migraines or marijuana intoxication (Simeon and Hollander 1993) as well as positive response to serotonin reuptake inhibitors (Fichtner et al. 1992; Hollander et al. 1990a).

■ Case 4: "A Stranger in the Mirror"—Depersonalization

A 28-year-old man developed chronic depersonalization symptoms after smoking marijuana 16 years previously. Symptoms included a sense of unreality, of detachment from the environment and his body, and of being "spaced out." Comorbid disorders included secondary depression, obsessive-compulsive personality disorder, and OCD characterized by aggressive obsessions and cleaning compulsions. Adequate trials of neuroleptics, tricyclics, MAOIs, and benzodiazepines failed to resolve the depersonalization. An infusion of intravenous methamphetamine 8 years after onset alleviated the symptoms for 30 minutes. Benzodiazepines reduced associated anxiety but not depersonalization symptoms. Clomipramine 400 mg/day yielded partial improvement in the OCD and depression but not the depersonalization. Fluvoxamine 300 mg/day resolved the depersonalization symptoms in 5 weeks. The obsessive-compulsive symptoms and depression also improved. These gains remained after 4 months of follow-up.

# Summary

The concept of the compulsive spectrum of disorders has considerable value for a better understanding of and in the treatment of a wide range of patients who were previously thought to be treatment refractory. Contrasts with the impulsive spectrum of disorders further elucidate this concept. In our discussion of the compulsive spectrum, we have considered dimensional and categorical approaches as well as diagnostic and phenomenological considerations. Major neurobiological findings that may characterize the compulsive spectrum include increased serotonergic tone and increased frontal lobe activity, whereas an opposite pattern may be demonstrated in impulsive disorders. We have also addressed the treatment of OCD and other compulsive disorders, with particular emphasis on serotonin reuptake inhibitors, behavior therapy, and the alternative augmentation strategies.

# References

American Psychiatric Association: Diagnostic and Statistical Manual of Mental Disorders, 4th Edition. Washington, DC, American Psychiatric Association, 1994

Aronowitz B, Hollander E, Mannuzza S, et al: Soft signs and familial transmission of obssessive-compulsive disorder. Poster presented at the 145th annual meeting of the American Psychiatric Association, Washington, DC, May 1992

Aronowitz B, Hollander E, DeCaria CM, et al: Neuropsychology of obsessive-compulsive disorder: preliminary findings. Neuropsychiatry, Neuropsychology, and Behavioral Neurology 7:81–86, 1994

Arora RC, Meltzer HY: Serotonergic measures in the brains of suicide victims: 5-HT2 binding sites in the frontal cortex of suicide victims and control subjects. Am J Psychiatry 146:730–736, 1989

Åsberg M, Träskman L, Thorén P: 5-HIAA in the cerebrospinal fluid: a biochemical suicide predictor? Arch Gen Psychiatry 33:1193–1197, 1976

Azrin NH, Nunn RG, Frantz SE: Treatment of hairpulling: a comparative study of habit reversal negative practice training. J Behav Ther Exp Psychiatry 11:13–20, 1980

Baxter LR Jr, Phelps ME, Mazziotta JC, et al: Local cerebral glucose metabolic rates in obsessive-compulsive disorder: a comparison with rates in unipolar depression and in normal controls. Arch Gen Psychiatry 44:211–218, 1987

Baxter LR Jr, Schwartz JM, Bergman KS, et al: Caudate glucose metabolic rate changes with both drug and behavior therapy for obsessive-compulsive disorder. Arch Gen Psychiatry 49:681–689, 1992

Behar D, Rapoport JL, Berg CJ, et al: Computerized tomography and neuropsychological test measures in adolescents with obsessive-compulsive disorder. Am J Psychiatry 41:363–369, 1984

Boone KB, Ananth J, Philpott L, et al: Neuropsychological characteristics of nondepressed adults with obsessive-compulsive disorder. Neuropsychiatry, Neuropsychology, and Behavioral Neurology 4:96–109, 1991

Bornstein RA, Yang V: Neuropsychological performance in medicated and unmedicated patients with Tourette's disorder. Am J Psychiatry 148:468–471, 1991

Buttinger K, Hollander E, Walsh BT: M-CPP challenges in anorexia nervosa. Paper presented in symposium at the 143th annual meeting of the American Psychiatric Association, New York, May 1990

Christensen KJ, Kim SW, Dysken MW, et al: Neuropsychological performance in obsessive-compulsive disorder. Biol Psychiatry 31:4–18, 1992

Christenson GA, Mackenzie TB, Mitchell JE: Characteristics of 60 adult chronic hair pullers. Am J Psychiatry 148:365–370, 1991

The Clomipramine Collaborative Study Group: Clomipramine in the treatment of patients with obsessive-compulsive disorder. Arch Gen Psychiatry 48:730–738, 1991

Coccaro EF, Siever LJ, Klar HM, et al: Serotonergic studies in affective and personality disorder patients: correlations with behavioral aggression and impulsivity. Arch Gen Psychiatry 46:587–599, 1989

Coccaro EF, Astill JL, Herbert JL, et al: Fluoxetine treatment of impulsive aggression in DSM-III-R personality disorder patients. J Clin Psychopharmacol 10:373–375, 1990

Cohen LJ, Hollander E, Badaracco MA: What the eyes can't see: diagnosis and treatment of somatic obsessions and delusions. Harvard Review of Psychiatry 2:160–165, 1994

Cohen LJ, Stein DJ, Simeon D, et al: Clinical profile, comorbidity, and treatment history in 123 hair pullers: a survey study. J Clin Psychiatry 56:319–326, 1995

Fallon BA, Rasmussen SA, Liebowitz MR: Hypochondriasis, in Obsessive-Compulsive–Related Disorders. Edited by Hollander E. Washington, DC, American Psychiatric Press, 1993, pp 71–92

Fichtner CG, Horevitz RP, Braun BG: Fluoxetine in depersonalization disorder. Am J Psychiatry 149:1750–1751, 1992

Flor-Henry P, Yeudall LT, Koles ZJ, et al: Neuropsychological and power spectral EEG investigations of the obsessive-compulsive syndrome. Biol Psychiatry 14:119–130, 1979

Foa EB, Steketee G: Obsessive-compulsive disorder, in Handbook of Phobia Therapy: Rapid Symptom Relief in Anxiety Disorders. Edited by Lindemann C. Northvale, NJ, Jason Aronson, 1989, pp 181–206

Goodman WK, Price LH, Rasmussen SA, et al: The Yale-Brown Obsessive Compulsive Scale, I: development, use, and reliability. Arch Gen Psychiatry 46:1006–1011, 1989a

Goodman WK, Price LH, Rasmussen SA, et al: The Yale-Brown Obsessive Compulsive Scale, II: validity. Arch Gen Psychiatry 46:1012–1016, 1989b

Goyer PF, Andreason PJ, Semple WE, et al: PET and personality disorders (abstract). Biol Psychiatry 29(9A):111 (94A), 1991

Head D, Bolton D, Hymas N: Deficits in cognitive shifting ability in patients with obsessive-compulsive disorder. Biol Psychiatry 25:929–937, 1989

Hoehn-Saric R, Pearlson GD, Harris CJ, et al: Effects of fluoxetine on regional cerebral blood flow in obsessive-compulsive patients. Am J Psychiatry 48:1243–1245, 1991

Hollander E: Introduction, in Obsessive-Compulsive–Related Disorders. Edited by Hollander E. Washington, DC, American Psychiatric Press, 1993a, pp 1–16

Hollander E: Obsessive-Compulsive–Related Disorders. Washington, DC, American Psychiatric Press, 1993b

Hollander E, Cohen LJ: Assessment and treatment of refractory anxiety. J Clin Psychiatry 55 (no 2, suppl):27–31, 1994

Hollander E, Liebowitz MR, Winchel R, et al: Treatment of body dysmorphic disorder with serotonin reuptake blockers. Am J Psychiatry 146:768–770, 1989

Hollander E, Liebowitz MR, DeCaria CM, et al: Treatment of depersonalization with serotonin reuptake blockers. J Clin Psychopharmacol 10:200–203, 1990a

Hollander E, Schiffman E, Cohen B, et al: Signs of central nervous system dysfunction in obsessive-compulsive disorder. Arch Gen Psychiatry 47:27–32, 1990b

Hollander E, DeCaria CM, Aronowitz B, et al: A pilot follow-up study of childhood soft signs and the development of adult psychopathology. Clinical and Research Reports 3(2):186–189, 1991a

Hollander E, DeCaria CM, Gully R, et al: Effects of chronic fluoxetine treatment on behavioral and neuroendocrine response to metachlorophenylpiperazine in obsessive-compulsive disorder. Psychiatry Res 36:1–17, 1991b

Hollander E, DeCaria CM, Saoud JB, et al: M-CPP activated regional cerebral blood flow in obsessive-compulsive disorder (abstract). Biol Psychiatry 29:280 (170A), 1991c

Hollander E, Liebowitz MR, Rosen WG: Neuropsychiatric and neuropsychological studies in obsessive-compulsive disorder, in The Psychobiology of Obsessive-Compulsive Disorder. Edited by Zohar J, Insel TR, Rasmussen SA. New York, Springer, 1991d, pp 126–145

Hollander E, Carrasco JL, Mullen LS, et al: Left hemispheric activation in depersonalization disorder: a case report. Biol Psychiatry 31:1157–1162, 1992a

Hollander E, Cohen LJ, DeCaria CM, et al: Fluoxetine and depersonalization syndrome (letter). Psychosomatics 33:361, 1992b

Hollander E, DeCaria CM, Nitescu A, et al: Serotonergic function in obsessive-compulsive disorder: behavioral and neuroendocrine responses to oral m-CPP and fenfluramine in patients and healthy volunteers. Arch Gen Psychiatry 49:21–28, 1992c

Hollander E, Frenkel M, DeCaria CM, et al: Treatment of pathological gambling with clomipramine (letter). Am J Psychiatry 149:710–711, 1992d

Hollander E, Cohen LJ, Simeon D: Body dysmorphic disorder. Psychiatric Annals 23:359–364, 1993a

Hollander E, Stein DJ, DeCaria CM, et al: A pilot study of biological predictors of treatment outcome in obsessive-compulsive disorder. Biol Psychiatry 33:747–749, 1993b

Hollander E, Stein DJ, DeCaria CM, et al: Serotonergic sensitivity in borderline personality disorder: preliminary findings. Am J Psychiatry 151:277–280, 1994

Insel TR: Toward a neuroanatomy of obsessive-compulsive disorder. Arch Gen Psychiatry 49:739–744, 1992

Insel TR, Mueller EA, Alterman I, et al: Obsessive-compulsive disorder and serotonin: is there a connection? Biol Psychiatry 20:1174–1188, 1985

Jenike MA, Baer L, Ballantine T, et al: Cingulotomy for refractory obsessive-compulsive disorder: a long-term follow-up of 33 patients. Arch Gen Psychiatry 48:548–555, 1991

Josephson SC, Brondolo E: Cognitive-behavioral approaches to obsessive-compulsive–related disorders, in Obsessive-Compulsive–Related Disorders. Edited by Hollander E. Washington, DC, American Psychiatric Press, 1993, pp 215–240

Kaye WH, Gwirtsman HE, George DT, et al: Altered serotonin activity in anorexia nervosa after long-term weight restoration: does elevated cerebrospinal fluid 5-hydroxyindoleacetic acid level correlate with rigid and obsessive behavior? Arch Gen Psychiatry 48:556–562, 1991

Linnoila M, Virkkunen M, Scheinen M, et al: Low cerebrospinal fluid 5-hydroxyindoleacetic acid concentration differentiates impulsive from nonimpulsive violent behavior. Life Sci 33:2609–2614, 1983

Martinot JL, Allilaire JF, Mazoyer BM, et al: Obsessive-compulsive disorder: a clinical, neuropsychological and positron emission tomography study. Acta Psychiatr Scand 82:233–242, 1990

Moffitt TE, Henry B: Neuropsychological studies of juvenile delinquency and violence: a review, in The Neuropsychology of Aggression. Edited by Milner J. Norwell, MA, Kluwer Academic, 1991, pp 67–91

Neziroglu FA, Yaryura-Tobias JA: Exposure, response prevention and cognitive therapy in the treatment of body dysmorphic disorder. Behavior Therapy 24:431–438, 1993

Phillips KA, McElroy SL, Keck PE Jr, et al: Body dysmorphic disorder: 30 cases of imagined ugliness. Am J Psychiatry 150:302–308, 1993

Pollard CA, Ibe IO, Krojanker DN, et al: Clomipramine treatment of trichotillomania: a follow-up report on four cases. J Clin Psychiatry 52:128–139, 1991

Quitkin F, Rifkin A, Klein DF: Neurological soft signs in schizophrenia and character disorders. Arch Gen Psychiatry 33:845–853, 1976

Rubin RT, Villanueva-Meyer J, Ananth J, et al: Regional xenon-133 cerebral blood flow and cerebral technetium Tc 99m-HMPAO uptake in unmedicated patients with obsessive-compulsive disorder and matched normal control subjects: determination by high-resolution single-photon emission computed tomography. Arch Gen Psychiatry 49:695–702, 1992

Shapiro AK, Shapiro ES: Treatment of tic disorders with haloperidol, in Tourette's Syndrome and Tic Disorders: Clinical Understanding and Treatment. Edited by Cohen DJ, Bruun RD, Leckman JF. New York, Wiley, 1988, pp 267–280

Simeon D, Hollander E: Depersonalization disorder. Psychiatric Annals 23:382–388, 1993

Stein DJ, Hollander E: Low-dose pimozide augmentation of serotonin reuptake blockers in the treatment of trichotillomania. J Clin Psychiatry 53:123–126, 1992

Stein DJ, Hollander E, Anthony DT, et al: Serotonergic medications for sexual obsessions, sexual addictions, and paraphilias. J Clin Psychiatry 53:267–271, 1992

Stein DJ, Hollander E, Chan S, et al: Computed tomography and neurological soft signs in obsessive-compulsive disorder. Psychiatry Res [Neuroimaging] 50:143–150, 1993a

Stein DJ, Hollander E, Cohen LJ, et al: Neuropsychiatric impairment in impulsive personality disorders. Psychiatry Res 48:257–266, 1993b

Stein DJ, Hollander E, Cohen LJ, et al: Serotonergic responsivity in trichotillomania: neuroendocrine effects of m-chlorophenylpiperazine. Biol Psychiatry (in press)

Swedo SE: Trichotillomania, in Obsessive-Compulsive–Related Disorders. Edited by Hollander E. Washington, DC, American Psychiatric Press, 1993a, pp 93–111

Swedo SE: Trichotillomania. Psychiatric Annals 23:402–407, 1993b

Swedo SE, Leonard HL: Trichotillomania: an obsessive-compulsive disorder? Psychiatr Clin North Am 15:777–790, 1992

Swedo SE, Leonard HL, Rapoport JL, et al: A double-blind comparison of clomipramine and desipramine in the treatment of trichotillomania (hair pulling). N Engl J Med 321:497–501, 1989

Swedo SE, Pietrini P, Leonard HL, et al: Cerebral glucose metabolism in childhood-onset obsessive-compulsive disorder: revisualization during pharmacotherapy. Arch Gen Psychiatry 49:690–694, 1992

Thorén P, Åsberg M, Bertilsson L, et al: Clomipramine treatment of obsessive-compulsive disorder, II: biochemical aspects. Arch Gen Psychiatry 37:1289–1294, 1980

Tupper DE: Soft Neurological Signs. Orlando, FL, Grune & Stratton, 1987

Valenstein ES: Great and Desperate Cures: The Rise and Decline of Psychosurgery and Other Radical Treatments for Mental Illness. New York, Basic Books, 1986

Yaryura-Tobias JA, Neziroglu F: Obsessive Compulsive Disorder: Pathogenesis, Diagnosis, and Treatment. New York, Marcel Dekker, 1983

Zielinski CM, Taylor MA, Juzwin KR: Neuropsychological deficits in obsessive-compulsive disorder. Neuropsychiatry, Neuropsychology, and Behavioral Neurology 4:110–126, 1991

Zohar J, Mueller EA, Insel TR, et al: Serotonergic responsivity in obsessive-compulsive disorder: comparison of patients and healthy controls. Arch Gen Psychiatry 44:946–951, 1987

Zohar J, Insel TR, Berman KF, et al: Anxiety and cerebral blood flow during behavioral challenge: dissociation of central from peripheral and subjective measures. Arch Gen Psychiatry 45:167–172, 1988

# 7

# Antianxiety Function of Impulsivity and Compulsivity

Susan C. Vaughan, M.D.
Leon Salzman, M.D.

In this chapter we present a psychoanalytic model of impulsivity and compulsivity. In this system, impulsive and compulsive symptoms are considered two potential end results of intrapsychic conflict. Intrapsychic conflict arises between unconscious drives and the forces that strive to contain their expression and/or between the various agencies (id, ego, superego) of the mind. When conflict is handled through compromises that partially satisfy the aims of each side in the struggle, the resultant behavior is adaptive and expresses aspects of the underlying conflict but no symptoms arise. However, when such a compromise formation cannot be reached, various types of symptomatic behavior occur. Impulsive behavior, whether as a single act or a defining character trait, suggests that the containing capacities of the ego are too weak relative to drive or affective states. In contrast, in compulsivity the ego is capable of containing impulses and modulating unpleasant affects. The symptoms of compulsivity represent a form of compromise, but the price paid for the impulse and affect modulation by the ego is loss of some normal function. The symptoms arise in the form of a repetitive symbolic act that gives a sense of pseudocontrol of impulses and affects at the expense of their modification into higher-order, subliminatory behaviors.

We first briefly review relevant analytic principles and then explore psychodynamic models of impulsivity and compulsivity and their relation to one another.

# Anxiety, Affects, and the
# Psychoanalytic Model of the Mind

An understanding of psychoanalytic perspectives on impulsivity and compulsivity requires a knowledge of three fundamental assumptions of the psychoanalytic model of the mind. First, a central hypothesis of psychoanalysis is the existence of the *dynamic unconscious,* which includes active instinctual drives and wishes, fantasies, and object representations. These unconscious contents press for behavioral expression but encounter opposition from other mental forces that seek to contain them within the unconscious.

Second, and closely allied with the idea of the dynamic unconscious, is the psychoanalytic belief that *intrapsychic conflict is pervasive and ubiquitously expressed in the thoughts, feelings, and behaviors of everyday life.* For example, a man with aggressive, angry feelings toward his boss may be 15 minutes late to an important business meeting because he took a wrong turn on the way to work on the very route that he has taken daily for years. He may then feel horrified and apologetic for the trouble that he has caused. His aggressive feelings toward his boss are thereby given a small outlet, while the intrapsychic forces that strive to contain his aggression are quickly mobilized and lead him to apologize profusely, covering up his aggressive feelings. Freud believed that all behaviors and feelings, including neurotic symptoms, are the result of such compromise formations. He noted that "neurotic symptoms are the outcome of a conflict. . . . The two forces which have fallen out meet once again in the symptom and are reconciled, as it were, by the compromise of the symptom that has been constructed. It is for that reason, too, that the symptom is so resistant: it is supported from both sides" (Freud 1917[1916–1917]/1963, pp. 358–359). Character, too, can be seen in part as the outcome of a conflict and consists of repeated, similar compromise formations across situations. Thus, the psychoanalytic model holds that some thoughts and behaviors in daily life are the derivatives of largely unconscious conflicts and reflect an intrapsychic balancing act, either between impulses and the defensive forces that restrain them or among the various agencies of the mind.

A third important assumption of the psychoanalytic model is the existence of *psychic determinism,* which posits that the connections between thoughts, feelings, and behaviors are not arbitrary. Rather, they are determined by and can be understood in terms of what came before them, even though the connecting links may not be readily apparent on initial inspection. Psychic determinism provides the rationale for the psychoanalytic technique of *free association.* When the patient reports whatever comes to mind without censoring his or her flow of associations, what emerges are the connecting links between ideas and feelings that act as signposts, pointing the way toward specific unconscious conflicts. Thus, by following the patient's associations, the analyst can elucidate the original intrapsychic conflict.

Intrapsychic conflict is also important because the conflict itself is believed to generate specific negative internal affect states, prominent among which may be anxiety and depression. Parenthetically, in working with clinical material, analysts stress the importance of following the patient's affect because it serves as a "royal road" to intrapsychic conflict and highlights places where smoothly functioning compromises have not been effected.

Anxiety is an affective state with a special place in the history of psychoanalysis and is particularly relevant to impulsivity and compulsivity. In Freud's first model of the mind, the *topographic model,* undischarged drives, particularly libidinal (sexual) drives, were hypothesized to cause anxiety. Thus, anxiety was the result of the repression of libido. However, in the *structural model,* which defined the ego, id, and superego as the agencies of the mind, the psychoanalytic understanding of anxiety shifted. Rather than being conceived of as arising from repressed libidinal drives, anxiety was seen as an affect that signaled to the ego the presence of psychic conflict. When external or intrapsychic events threaten to resurrect unresolved unconscious conflicts, the anxiety generated signals the ego to mobilize its defenses. The defenses effect a compromise formation between the competing forces of the mind, one that permits each of the conflicting drives or structures some degree of expression. If defenses operate efficiently, they reduce anxiety by warding off the emergence of the conflict into consciousness. Over time, successfully operating defenses become rigidified into what Reich (1933/1945) termed "character armor," a personality-defining style of defensive operations. Alternatively, the mobilization of defenses may fail, which would lead to symptom formation. In this case, the symptoms themselves bear the mark of the defensive conflict from which they originate. As Freud (1896/1962) stated regarding compulsive thoughts, the return of the repressed memory or conflict comes about in the distorted form of obsessive ideas which constitute "structures in the nature of a *compromise* between the repressed ideas and the repressing ones" (p. 170). (See discussions by Brenner [1973, 1982] and Arlow and Brenner [1964] for a fuller overview of the fundamental assumptions of the psychoanalytic model of the mind, the topographical and structural theories, and the role of affects and anxiety.)

# Impulsivity

Impulsivity, whether a circumscribed symptom or a character-defining pattern of behavior, can be seen in psychoanalytic terms in three ways, stemming from original drive theory, structural theory, and object relations models. In drive theory terms, impulsivity is seen as the welling up of a drive that leads to sudden, sometimes explosive, unpremeditated actions. The resultant behavior feels irresistible to the person experiencing it and is accompanied by the reduction of the original drive state. In this way, impulsive behaviors are seen as the relatively undistorted expression of primary drives. They often have a clearly gratifying quality in the moment of action in that they satisfy the push for expression of sexual and aggressive drives. The relatively unmodified and pleasurable nature of the drive and of its expression tends to give the impulsive behavior an understandable quality to the outside observer. This is in contrast to checking and other ritualistic behaviors of the compulsive person that often have a bizarre and incomprehensible quality (Frosch et al. 1993). Thus, a person who, in a moment of blind rage, throttles someone with whom he or she is angry is gratifying his or her aggressive impulse in a relatively unmodified form in a way that feels ego-syntonic at the moment of action, even though he or she may later feel remorse. The motive, or drive, behind the impulsive act is understandable to an observer. In the drive theory model, the discharge of drives through impulsive behavior actually gives rise to ego weakness, because psychic energy is discharged and therefore not available to fuel higher subliminatory behaviors. Thus, ego weakness is self-reinforcing; a weak ego cannot contain the drive and also cannot harness the energy behind the drive for more-modified, less-impulsive behavioral pursuits. The man who attacks someone when he is angry may be unable to contain his aggressive impulses adequately to make, for example, a successful football player; he may go to jail rather than to the Super Bowl.

Although drives remain important in modern psychoanalytic thought, behaviors are rarely characterized purely in terms of Freud's original drive theory. A more typical and modern psychoanalytic view would be to cast impulsive behavior within the framework of the structural model. In this model, affects, including anxiety, arise because of conflicts between the agencies of the mind, often between the id and ego or superego. Impulsive behavior occurs when negative affective states such as anxiety generated by intrapsychic conflict become unbearable and need to be dissipated. Thus, an intolerable affect of anxiety generated during a conflict with another person may be dissipated by impulsively lashing out. In the structural model, there are differences between individuals in the relative role of ego versus superego weakness in the genesis of impulsive behaviors. The person with superego weakness may justify his or her assault of another person with rationalizations and will not feel ashamed after the attack, whereas the individual with an intact superego who is impulsive because of ego weakness will experience shame and guilt following the expression of an impulse. Jail is a form of societal imposition of external superego controls for the person who lacks an internally based conscience.

The structural model may also be used to examine impulsive behaviors that are directed toward the self. For example, a patient in whom ego weakness predominates may feel an urge to impulsively drink until intoxicated. This urge may be experienced as irresistible but does not clearly gratify a primary libidinal or aggressive impulse. Rather, it dissipates a feeling of anxiety and is pleasurable specifically because it relieves this intolerable state. It may not be readily understandable to an outside observer why the person is drinking; the alcohol is an external way of achieving the anxiolytic effect that in another person might be handled through the ego's own internal modulatory mechanisms. If the ego was functioning well, it could mobilize the defenses needed to repress fully the unconscious conflict, thereby reducing the signal anxiety produced by the emergence of the conflict.

The object relations model, the most modern of the three psychoanalytic theoretical frames, arises naturally from structural theory and sheds light on the role of identification in ego and superego formation. Early relationships (object relations) with caretakers are internalized during maturation by children. The process of internalization consists first of imitation of significant others followed by introjection, in which all aspects of the object (caretaker) are taken in and internally represented. Finally, this introjection of the whole object is modified to identification with important parts of the parent. With the development of identification, a child can be like the parent in important ways without being like him or her in every way. These early object representations of relationships with significant others are the building blocks from which the ego is formed. The ego-ideal is a coalescence of these early object representations that, in combination with the internalization of external parental controls, gives rise to the superego.

In the object relations model, impulsivity occurs because of a failure of ego or superego development with resultant ego or superego weakness. Ego weakness arises when conflicting internal representations of self and others are not integrated during development. Fairbairn (1954, 1963) proposed an object relations theory of ego development in which aggressive drives are viewed as a reaction to frustration and deprivation by caretakers. In creating an internalized representation of others, the infant incorporates both the gratifying and the frustrating aspects of the person but keeps the two separate. Eventually, during the course of normal development, these two split internal representations are integrated into a cohesive object representation that becomes a building block for the ego. Kernberg (1975, 1976) proposed that when frustration predominates in the infant's early experiences with caretakers, the aggressive drives become stronger and inhibit the ability of the developing infant to integrate the split-off good and bad representations of self and others. In his model, when frustration predominates, the intensity of negative affect attached to bad object representations threatens to overwhelm and annihilate good internal objects. Thus, the developing infant is left with permanently split (good vs. bad) representations of self and other, which sets the stage for future use of primitive defenses such as idealization, devaluation, and splitting by a weak, unintegrated ego. This is Kernberg's proposed pathogenesis of what he has termed "borderline personality organization," in which the use of these defensive maneuvers leads to low anxiety tolerance and poor impulse control.

Winnicott (1960/1965, 1965) further highlighted the importance of early object relations in ego development, proposing that a "good-enough mother" will achieve an optimal balance of gratification and frustration of the infant's needs, thereby creating a suitable holding environment for ego development. The inevitable frustration of the infant, whose needs cannot be immediately and perfectly met by the mother the instant they arise, is believed in this model to create an internal push for ego growth and development. Such frustration creates an impetus for self-regulation and the mastery of negative internal states and drive frustrations on the part of the infant. Frosch (1977) suggested that the infant's prior experiences of gratification lead to an ability to anticipate that his or her needs will ultimately be met. This ability to anticipate gratification based on past experience actually serves to decrease the intensity of internal tensions and thereby furthers the capacity for tolerance of delay. In a way, this can be viewed as the opposite of anticipatory anxiety; anticipatory gratification can serve as a way of self-regulating affective states. This model also suggests that overgratification of the infant's every need hinders the development of that optimal level of frustration that, under normal circumstances, spurs proper ego development. In an atmosphere of (continual) overgratification, the child's potential for developing the capacity to delay gratification is not realized and indeed may wither, leaving the child without the capacity to either bear anxiety-inducing situations or to tolerate related negative affects.

Because the superego is felt to arise from the ego, faulty ego development as well as identification with and imitation of parents with superego pathology can lead to superego weakness. Further, caretakers who provide inadequate external controls for children during development set the stage for the child to have problems in the internalization of externally imposed controls that lead to self-control. (See Sandler 1960 and Sandler et al. 1963 for more detailed discussion of the ego-ideal and development of the superego.)

In reality, these three contrasting models of impulsivity are intertwined, and impulsive behavior may serve more than one function. Zetzel (née Rosenberg 1949) noted that anxiety arises both from frustrated, undischarged drive tension and in response to the mobilization of internal danger in the form of conflict. In fact, a single act can often represent the discharge of a primary libidinal or aggressive drive, the modification of an affective state such as anxiety, and an enactment of an important object relation that has been internalized. For example, when someone feels an impulse to masturbate in response to the welling up of a sexual drive, the masturbation can be seen as the immediate expression of the drive and as a response to an anxious internal state that will be dissipated or soothed by self-stimulation and orgasm. Further, if the sexual drive predominantly takes the form of masturbation rather than sexual intimacy with a partner, this may suggest problems in early object relationships that resulted in impaired capacity for intimacy in adult life.

Psychoanalytic theory also recognizes that impulsive acts can result from a relative imbalance between the strength of the impulses and affects and the ego's ability to contain and modulate them. There is evidence that neonates have striking variations in their response to frustration (Thomas et al. 1963). Such individual differences in temperament are the biological substrate in which object relations and ego/superego development occur. Those with strong inborn responses to frustration may be at a disadvantage in that they must develop relatively stronger defenses and ego strength to contain and modify their drives. Also, strong negative responses to frustration may adversely impact relationships with caretakers, who may perceive the infant as too demanding or difficult.

In later life, the emergence of a syndrome such as an anxiety disorder may tip the balance between drives or affects and relative ego strength in the direction of impulsive action. For example, a patient with panic attacks and generalized anxiety disorder attempted to modulate his uncomfortable, anxious internal states through frequent and time-consuming masturbation that was markedly increased from his normal pattern. During masturbation and briefly following ejaculation, the patient experienced a diminution in his anxiety. It is noteworthy that the patient's impulse to masturbate, seemingly driven on each occasion by intolerable anxiety, became, as it was repeatedly enacted, a compulsion. This example highlights the interesting interplay between impulsive drives and compulsive behaviors. When the patient's panic and anxiety were treated with a tricyclic antidepressant and a benzodiazepine, the impulsive push that the patient felt to masturbate returned to baseline. Psychoanalytic theory increasingly appreciates the role of factors such as inborn temperamental differences in aggressive drives and affective dysregulation as determinants of impulsive behavior.

Kernberg's concept of borderline personality organization, which incorporates elements of drive theory, structural theory, and object relations, provides a unifying framework for examining patients with impulse-ridden personalities. For example, one patient met Kernberg's criteria for borderline personality organization, including 1) identity diffusion, which is a lack of integration of the internal representation of self and others; 2) predominant use of primitive defense mechanisms such as denial, projective identification, splitting, and omnipotent control; and 3) an intact capacity for reality testing, which distinguishes borderline from psychotic personality organization. Following a disagreement with a nurse regarding her medication, the patient smashed a large plate-glass window in the nursing station. After discussion of the incident in exploratory psychotherapy, it seemed a plausible hypothesis that the behavior both discharged a primary aggressive drive and dissipated an intolerable internal sense of badness and anxiety. In addition, it was an enactment of a sadomasochistic object relation that had occurred in childhood with her abusive, alcoholic mother. In this enactment, the patient responded to the nurse's attempt to get her to take medication by assuming the role of the frightening, out-of-control sadistic mother. At other points, this patient's impulsive cutting of herself seemed primarily designed to eliminate a sense of internal emptiness that was accompanied by anxiety rather than to discharge any primary libidinal or aggressive drive. Her impulsive difficulties might be understood within a psychodynamic framework to indicate that she had exceptionally strong inborn drives and affects; she had a history of colic and was noted to be difficult to console and soothe in infancy by several relatives. However, it is difficult to describe and quantify excessive inborn aggression in an objective fashion. Alternatively, her impulsivity can be understood as arising from a weak ego whose development was stunted by a depriving and frustratingly neglectful alcoholic mother and, in the case of smashing the window, as an enactment of this primary object relation with the nurse. Further, excessive aggression, ego weakness, and faulty early object relations can be interrelated; the infant may be perceived as too demanding by a mother with impaired frustration tolerance herself, resulting in maternal abuse and neglect that in turn generates increased aggression and decreased capacity for self-modulation in the infant. (See Stone 1988 for an overview of these issues in borderline personality disorder.)

Thus, in psychoanalytic terms, both single impulsive acts and the impulsive character pathology evident in those persons with borderline personality organization can be seen as a mismatch between opposing drives or affective states that push for expression or modulation and the capacity of the ego to modify and contain them. This psychoanalytic view of a unified spectrum of impulsive behavior is in contrast to the categorical classification system of DSM-IV (American Psychiatric Association 1994). In DSM-IV, syndromes of impulse dyscontrol such as pyromania, kleptomania, intermittent explosive disorder, and pathological gambling are classified on Axis I, whereas personality disorders in which impulsivity may be a prominent feature are classified on Axis II. Impulsivity resulting from borderline personality organization can be an important feature in a number of Axis II syndromes, including DSM-IV borderline, paranoid, schizoid, narcissistic, histrionic, and antisocial personality disorders. Further, the structural organization of other personality disorders such as avoidant, dependent, and passive-aggressive, as defined within the DSM classification system, remains equivocal (Oldham et al. 1985). With the redefinition of histrionic personality disorder in DSM-III-R (American Psychiatric Association 1987) and DSM-IV, it is less likely that patients meeting the criteria for this disorder will have borderline personality organization (Kernberg 1985).

Kernberg's model also provides a unifying framework for examining many personality types previously defined by analysts in which impulsivity is a prominent feature, such as Deutsch's (1942) "as if " characters, Zetzel's (1968) type 3 and 4 histrionic characters, and so-called hysteroid dysphoric and infantile characters (Klein 1977). (See Greenberg and Mitchell 1983 and Sutherland 1980 for a more in-depth discussion of the underpinnings of these object relations models.)

Further, many behaviors that are termed "impulsive" in the current classification system are behaviors that are considered "bad," for the individual, for those around him or her, or for society as a whole. In contrast, psychoanalytic theory does not make a sharp distinction between various types of impulsivity but sees all impulsive behaviors on a spectrum. Impulsive behaviors are not considered "bad" in superego terms. Rather, they are seen as a means of discharging drives, negative internal affective states such as anxiety resulting from internal conflict, or both.

Whether it occurs as a limited symptom or a character-defining trait, impulsivity has been considered to suggest a poor prognosis and to interfere with psychoanalytic treatment (Lansky 1989). Psychoanalytic treatments are based on the patient's having a reasonable capacity for reporting thoughts, feelings, and fantasies in a verbal form during sessions, which revolve around the working-through of conflicts between impulses and the defenses against them. In addition, the procedure, particularly in psychoanalysis, requires a reasonable capacity to delay action and to speak about rather than enact impulses. The relatively inactive listening position of the analyst may be experienced by patients as withholding or depriving, particularly as the patient regresses in the analytic situation. These characteristics of the treatment situation often make it more difficult for patients with impulsivity to tolerate psychoanalytic treatments.

However, it is interesting to note that Freud (1914/1958) rapidly recognized that many important communications from the patient were not remembered and verbally reported but rather were repeated in action. In "Remembering, Repeating and Working-Through," Freud acknowledged that conflicts could be put into action rather than words. Acting out for a patient in an analysis may consist of using behavior as a defensive maneuver that anticipates the emergence of a conflict. For example, a patient may repeatedly come late to sessions as a way to regulate the amount of session time left to address his or her angry feelings toward the therapist. In this case, an investigation of the lateness may lead to increased understanding of the patient's aggressive fantasies and fears about expressing them. Thus, the behavior itself might serve an important communicative function. In contrast, a more impulsive patient who becomes angry with the therapist in a session may storm out of the room, ending the hour. In this case, the impulsivity is a response to the emergence of a conflict rather than an anticipation of its emergence. The response of walking out may contain little information that is helpful in understanding the conflict. Rather than being an information-rich enactment of an unconscious fantasy or the defense against it, impulsivity in the therapeutic situation often simply represents the best available response to conflict or frightening affect of a momentarily overloaded ego.

Recent modifications of classical psychoanalytic technique, such as that proposed by Kernberg (1984; Kernberg et al. 1990) for patients with impulsive, borderline-level character organization, involve both supportive and expressive techniques and the use of parameters such as treatment contracts and limit setting regarding acting out. For example, a patient who makes an impulsive suicide attempt and then phones the analyst to report the behavior rather than immediately seeking medical attention might be terminated from treatment because he violated a fundamental tenet of the treatment contract. This technique of forcing the patient to accept responsibility for his impulsive gestures helps to tilt the balance within the therapy in the direction of verbal rather than behavioral expression of drives and negative affects, resulting in strengthening of the ego. Still, even with these modifications, the treatment of impulsive behaviors with psychodynamic therapies remains difficult because of the fundamental ego deficits that impulsivity implies.

# Compulsivity

Whereas in the impulsive patient a drive or affective state escapes the capacity of the ego to contain and modulate it, in the compulsive patient the ego attempts to contain the drive or affect. Intrapsychic conflict produces anxiety that signals the ego to mobilize its defenses. However, rather than the conflict being fully repressed and partial expression of each side of it being permitted in the form of a compromise formation, compulsive symptoms are formed. These symptoms are a result of the intensity of intrapsychic conflict relative to ego defenses. Compulsive symptoms arise through the action of certain typical defense mechanisms that the ego uses unsuccessfully to try to fully repress the conflict.

Freud's famous case of the "Rat Man," Paul Lorenz, illustrates these concepts in a clinical context. Freud first described this case and his ideas about obsessive pathology in "Notes Upon a Case of Obsessional Neurosis" (Freud 1909/1955). In this paper, Freud reported on the treatment of a 30-year-old lawyer who was plagued for 4 years by increasingly severe obsessional thoughts of rats boring into the anus and through the intestines of his father, who was deceased. This symptom can be understood as an expression both of the patient's aggressive impulses toward his father (in the form of death wishes) and of his fear of the consequences of these wishes (that his thoughts may have caused his father's death). The partially repressed conflict resulted in recurrent symptomatic compulsive thoughts (also termed *obsessions*) about the rat torture that were accompanied by tremendous anxiety. The anxiety is both a continuing signal that attempts to invoke the ego to repress the conflict through defensive operations and a result of the ego's failure to do so.

Freud initially focused on repression as the maneuver that begins all sequences of defensive operations. He then highlighted several typical defensive strategies that the ego of the compulsive individual uses to attempt to effect a compromise formation. These defense mechanisms include isolation of affect, undoing, overvaluation of thought, and reaction formation.

In *isolation of affect,* thoughts become disconnected from their associated affects. Previously unacceptable thoughts that are then "stripped of self reproach" emerge into consciousness. The affect dissociated from these thoughts becomes attached (i.e., "falsely connected") to another idea. Thus, in the case of the Rat Man, the affect of self-reproach or guilt became dissociated from the death wish for the father and attached to the idea of the rat torture, which is a derivative of the original wish in somewhat disguised form.

Further, the ego uses the defense of *undoing,* in which the aggressive wish is expressed and then taken back or undone through some ritualized thought or behavior. In a case such as the Rat Man's, the expression of the aggressive thought toward the father might be accompanied by a compulsive behavior such as checking to reassure himself that the imagined harm to the father has not actually transpired. Alternatively, the Rat Man might have an obsessional, undoing thought—such as "I was a loving and loyal son"—that follows that rat torture thought and neutralizes it.

Freud also highlighted the *overvaluation of thought* in the case of the Rat Man, stressing the patient's experience of his thoughts as extremely powerful, omnipotent wishes that were the equivalent of deeds. To the Rat Man, there was little difference between wishing his father dead and killing him.

*Reaction formation,* which involves a transformation of affects into their opposites, is a fourth typical defensive strategy with which obsessive-compulsive persons try to manage intrapsychic conflicts. In terms of the Rat Man, this might mean he would think, "I do not want to see my father tortured like this; I am only interested in ensuring that it doesn't happen."

The Rat Man's symptoms can also be seen as overdetermined, meaning that they fulfill multiple intrapsychic needs or goals simultaneously. The first thoughts of the rat torture occurred when the patient was talking to a cruel army captain who probably reminded him of earlier interactions with a tyrannical father whom he admired, hated, and feared and who had control over him.

Compulsive behaviors may be part of specific syndromes, as in Freud's "obsessional neurosis," now called obsessive-compulsive disorder (OCD) in DSM-IV terms. In addition, compulsive behaviors may be characteristic of a patient's overall personality style, as in Freud's early description (1908/1959) of the anal character, which was typified by the triad of orderliness, parsimoniousness, and obstinacy. This anal character style corresponds to obsessive-compulsive personality disorder (OCPD) in DSM-IV. In early analytic models, OCPD was felt to degenerate into and to be a prerequisite for OCD. Both disorders were believed to result from a regression to an anal-sadistic phase of psychosexual development. This regression was hypothesized to lead to the development of a harsh superego and to be prompted by precocious ego development that outstripped libidinal development. A historical perspective on the emergence of this original view has been detailed by Nagera (1976).

Recently, three important findings have resulted in a change in the analytic view of OCD and OCPD as being on a spectrum of different severity but with identical underlying psychodynamic mechanisms. First, there is now strong evidence that OCD and OCPD are not related to each other in the way analysts since Freud have assumed. Several more recent studies (Baer and Jenike 1992; Joffee et al. 1988; Pitman and Jenike 1989; Pollak 1987b) have provided evidence that OCPD is found only in a minority of patients with OCD. OCPD was less common than dependent, avoidant, and histrionic personality disorders in those with OCD. This does not mean that the two disorders may not coexist or be interrelated in some patients, as Munich (1986) has suggested in an interesting case report. He described the emergence of OCD symptoms during psychoanalysis in a patient with OCPD that were heralded by the emergence of preoedipal issues focused on loss and separation.

Second, biological evidence has emerged that points strongly toward neurological dysfunction in the caudate nucleus in OCD. This abnormality may give rise to faulty gating and screening of sensations, thoughts, and motor behaviors that are normally effectively inhibited by subcortical areas (Thompson et al. 1992). In this model, the presumably meaningful dynamic content of patient symptoms may, instead, reflect the dysfunction of the caudate nucleus rather than represent intrapsychic conflict. Put differently, the dynamic content of symptoms may represent the attachment of meaning to internal experiences that arise from brain dysfunction. Analysts have long stressed the idea that compulsive symptoms are the result of higher-level cortical functioning—ego mechanisms working to contain unconscious forces arising from subcortical aspects of the brain. This is in distinct contrast to the neurobiological view that the symptoms arise from impaired subcortical brain that impacts the cortex. Katz (1991) has attempted to integrate the two by suggesting that this subcortical, serotonergically mediated neurological impairment parallels the classic Freudian description of "failure of repression" in OCD. Gabbard (1992) asserts that dynamic principles are often useful in informing the treatment of those with OCD even though the intrapsychic conflicts that are often seemingly evident in the content of specific symptoms are no longer considered the primary cause of the disorder.

Third, in addition to the emergence of these biological data, many analysts now acknowledge that psychodynamic psychotherapy and analysis have been less than highly effective in the treatment of those with OCD (Esman 1989). Failure of psychodynamic treatment, the development of effective somatic therapies, and the discovery of underlying brain disease have influenced analytic perspectives on OCD. Although many years ago some analysts considered OCD a "brain disease," these findings have prompted other analysts to question their formulation of the disorder in terms of intrapsychic conflict alone.

In contrast, OCPD represents a personality type in which compulsivity is a key feature. Its description has remained remarkably constant since Freud's delineation of the anal character; in fact, all three features of Freud's anal character are reflected in the DSM-IV criteria for the disorder, and there is remarkable overlap and constancy between various classification systems (Pfohl and Blum 1991). A composite "compulsive character" profile was sketched by Pollak (1987a, pp. 249–250), who emphasized the personality as "cheerless and sober," "hard working," and attentive to detail to the point of rigidity and unspontaneous pedantry. Their preoccupation with order, efficiency, and strict adherence to rules makes persons with this personality perfectionistic and driven, and they often appear to be in a hurry and harassed by unending obligations and responsibility as they make unending attempts to attain order and perfection. Their self-image is that "of a conscientious, . . . responsible, [and] cautious" individual with "high, if not exacting, standards for self and others." However, these same traits may be experienced by others as rigid, stubborn, controlling and formal. Relations with others may be perceived largely "in terms of patterns of dominance and submission," and the obsessive individual is often secretly derisive of those who appear more emotionally expressive or vulnerable or impulsive.

In psychoanalytic terms, OCPD is still understood as the character that results from the typical ego defensive strategies of isolation of affect, undoing, overvaluation of thought, and reaction formation. However, more recent analytic writers have tended to emphasize one characteristic of the personality that they see as central. For example, Salzman (1968, 1980) stressed that the compulsive person's need for control in all aspects of life is a way of preventing feelings or thoughts that might be shame producing or give rise to loss of pride or status. In Salzman's model, the person with a compulsive personality has the constant sense of being in danger of falling short of the expectations of others. Such a person is constantly striving for approval and craves warm feelings from others and yet has difficulty expressing tender feelings to others and experiencing them in himself or herself. For example, a patient with OCPD might become tearful rather diffusely when experiencing any strong affect rather than specifically in response to sadness. In contrast, Rado (1974) highlighted the importance of power struggles and excessive rage, and MacKinnon and Michels (1971) viewed the core conflict in OCPD as an ongoing battle between obedience and defiance, particularly over issues of "time, money and dirt." These authors emphasized the continuous alternation between fear and rage typical of the compulsive personality. Shapiro (1965, 1981) examined the cognitive style of the obsessive person, a style that he believed was dominated by the thought "I should." Pointing to the compulsive person's excessive devotion to work, he also concluded that the obsessive person approaches play as if it were work, determined to have a good time. Shapiro saw this rigid cognitive style as a way to minimize doubt and rumination.

Mollinger (1980) proposed that, in fact, a marked antithetical quality pervades all compulsive personality styles. He noted that

> the major defense mechanisms of undoing, isolation and reaction formation all involve opposites: contradictory acts following each other, the keeping apart of ambivalent feeling states and the turning of wishes into their opposites. The cog-

nitive modes of the obsessive-compulsive are marked by dichotomies: sharply focused attention which misses essential points and a non-inclusive all-inclusiveness. The obsessive's regression to the anal phase produces ambivalent emotions, contradictory attitudes. . . . a harsh superego creates an alternation between obedience to it and defiance and feelings of both perfection and imperfection. (p. 475)

The question of why a person would develop a compulsive rather than, for example, a hysterical defensive style has also been a subject of psychoanalytic discourse. Early emphasis on "the battle of the chamber pot," the role of toilet-training experiences, and the regression to anal sadism in the etiology of compulsivity has shifted to an appreciation for the widespread struggles inherent in the developmental task of achieving autonomy and separation-individuation. A number of authors have highlighted the role of authoritarian, overcontrolling, probably obsessive parents in shaping the child's emphasis on issues of control. For example, Ingram (1982) suggested that the emphasis on control represents identification with the parent, and Lidz (1979) hypothesized that the parents' own inability to tolerate drives leads them to teach the child obsessive defenses as means of handling his or her aggressive and sexual drives. He points out "these obsessional parents . . . would almost certainly seek to limit the young child's autonomy . . . in many ways other than through bowel training" (p. 161). The idea that obsessive parents raise obsessive children is probably statistically likely given the widespread prevalence of the compulsive character type. The prevalence of compulsivity as a character trait that shades into a personality disorder probably reflects the fact that it is generally a quite adaptive coping strategy in industrialized, individualistic, and work-centered societies. However, compulsive personality can cause significant impairment in interpersonal functioning and is also associated with high rates of depressive disorders (Kaplan 1987).

In terms of structural theory and object relations, compulsivity can result from an overly harsh, punitive superego that is a composite of the ego-ideal formed from early object relations and the internalization of external controls imposed by early caretakers. In the patient with a harsh superego, any negative impulses, feelings, or thoughts are entirely unacceptable and must be completely eradicated. A harsh, perfectionistic parent with OCPD may transmit to a child an unrealistic ego-ideal that is impossible to live up to as well as a harsh set of rules about what constitutes acceptable thoughts, feelings, and behaviors. The child who imitates, incorporates, and ultimately identifies with a parent with OCPD is likely to have a superego that gives rise to the behaviors of OCPD.

Compulsivity, in contrast to impulsivity, was felt, even by Freud, to be quite amenable to psychoanalytic treatment. This was perhaps assumed because the dynamics of the condition are often readily apparent to an observer. As noted above, analytic treatments are not widely felt to be efficacious for OCD. However, long-term psychodynamic psychotherapy and psychoanalysis remain widely used mainstays of treatment for OCPD. In such treatments, those with OCPD may make impressive gains in understanding their fears and wishes and seeing how they use particular defensive maneuvers to avoid internal discomfort. However, it is noteworthy that many of these defensive maneuvers are quite ego-syntonic and that the intellectualizing defenses of the person with OCPD are often used as powerful resistances in the treatment and necessitate an active, confrontive approach on the part of the analyst or therapist (Salzman 1980). The psychoanalytic treatment of OCPD is often a long, slow process. There is no solid empirical evidence regarding the degree to which psychodynamic treatments are efficacious in OCPD. However, there are no other available treatment modalities for OCPD that have been shown to be efficacious or superior to psychodynamic therapies (Oldham and Frosch 1985).

# Relationship Between
# Impulsivity and Compulsivity

In contrast to biological models that may see impulsivity and compulsivity as disorders at polar ends of the serotonergic axis, both of which are moved toward normality through pharmacological intervention, psychoanalytic models would suggest a closer and less-polar relationship between the two. Depending on the strength of the drive to be discharged or the amount of anxiety generated by intrapsychic conflict to be contained and the relative ego strength of the person in that moment, anxiety/affective states and impulses can be contained through compulsive mechanisms or can overwhelm the capacity of the ego entirely and result in impulsivity. In a sense, compulsivity can be seen as a particular pattern of defensive maneuvers in a person with a strong ego in response to libidinal and aggressive drives or intolerable affects. In an individual with a weaker ego, these drives or affects might be dealt with through impulsivity. Superego functioning in impulsivity and compulsivity is variable but intertwined in important ways with ego functions. Impulsivity can occur in the setting of superego weakness, in which case the person experiences no remorse about impulsive behaviors that negatively impact others. In the impulsive patient with an intact superego, impulsive acts are often followed by shame and distress. Compulsive patients with ego weakness that gives rise to symptom formation are likely to have harsh, punitive superegos because of identification with perfectionistic parents who may themselves have OCPD. At best, when allowing themselves pleasures such as vacations, these persons will feel that they have "paid in advance" through hard work and self-deprivation.

It is also possible in this model that the same individual might exhibit impulsive and compulsive behaviors at different times depending on the intensity of the internal drives or affective states and the relative strength of the ego in those moments. Interplay between impulsivity and compulsivity has been described in several recent case reports, including Krueger's (1988) case studies of compulsive shopping and Wurmser's (1985) reports of compulsive drug use in patients with impulse-ridden character structures. These authors highlight that the repetitive impulsive behaviors of these patients have a compulsive quality.

To extend this view of the relationship between impulsivity and compulsivity, psychoanalytic theory holds that "normal" human behavior always involves an attempt to balance the push toward expression of drives with the defensive forces holding back the unbridled expression of these drives. Thus, even in the healthy individual, there are muted reflections of the pervasive, underlying struggle to achieve this balance. Impulsivity may be replaced by normal and desirable spontaneity in persons with egos strong enough to use mature defensive operations such as sublimation.

In sublimation, a compromise formation is reached and the original conflict, with its associated affect, is effectively managed by the ego. The result is a creative, transmuted expression of the original impulse in a socially acceptable, even admirable, manner. In part, this modification of the original impulse is made possible by frustration tolerance and the capacity for delay.

A form of desirable compulsivity is also present in successfully functioning individuals with the traits of carefulness and thoroughness. However, in contrast to the compulsivity of OCPD, the carefulness and thoroughness in these individuals can be seen as an attempt to achieve mastery over the tasks of one's daily life through practice. Thus, these traits require more flexibility and a tolerance for less pseudocontrol than is present in compulsivity.

Analysts believe that one needs drive discharge for optimal sexual functioning, creativity, a good sense of humor, and pleasurable affective connection with others. In addition, one needs appropriate muting of drive discharge for self-protection and subliminatory behaviors that depend on the ability to delay gratification. Thus, "normal" impulsivity and compulsivity are the yin and yang that reflect the operation of the opposing forces of the dynamic unconscious.

An echo of this psychoanalytic view can be seen in the work of Cloninger and his group (Cloninger et al. 1993; Svrakic et al. 1993), which is discussed in more detail in Chapter 3 of the present volume. Cloninger's model of personality defines three dimensions of temperament that together form the matrix for normal personality development. When a person's behavior lies at an extreme end of one of the three axes, it represents a personality disorder. However, Cloninger's model provides for much variation in combinations of the three axes that fall within the normal range.

Two specific axes seem particularly relevant to impulsivity and compulsivity. Novelty seeking, a heritable bias in the activation or initiation of behaviors, may be related to psychoanalytic concepts of impulsivity. In contrast, Cloninger's concept of harm avoidance, a temperamental factor that modulates inhibition or cessation of behaviors, may inform psychoanalytic descriptions of compulsivity. Specific biological factors such as temperament are the biological substrate in which ego development and early object relations un-fold and may therefore also determine the propensity of individuals for particular defensive styles.

# Conclusions

The psychoanalytic view of impulsivity and compulsivity sees these behaviors as two different modalities for dealing with intrapsychic conflict. The two are conceptualized as being on a spectrum from 1) impulsive symptoms that reflect relative ego weakness to 2) compulsive symptoms that reflect enough ego strength to contain drives and affects but not enough to effect successful conflict resolution to 3) normal adaptive functioning that results from successful compromise formation. In addition to ego strength, the superego plays an important role in determining whether impulsive and compulsive behaviors provoke guilt and shame or rationalization. Impulsive behaviors reflect a relative imbalance between intrapsychic conflict and the overwhelming push for drive discharge, the affective modulation that the drive discharge produces, and the ego's containing and modulating capacities. Compulsive behaviors reflect the use of rigid and character-defining defense mechanisms that strain to successfully contain drives and ward off negative affects but are unable to achieve completely effective compromise formations.

In contrast, when a person's ego is strong and functions well, the ubiquitous, ongoing conflicts that arise within the dynamic unconscious are settled by compromise formations without reaching conscious awareness or resulting in symptom formation. The thoughts, conscious fantasies, feelings, and behaviors of daily life bear the mark of the original conflicts but represent adaptive functioning. Some drive expression occurs as well as some representation of defenses in the resultant behavior; the person can enjoy appetitive drives and their gratification, has a capacity for spontaneity but also an ability to delay gratification and to engage in subliminatory behaviors, and has an ability to thoughtfully reflect before acting.

The psychoanalytic notion that impulsivity and compulsivity are two ways to deal with intrapsychic conflict that are on a spectrum depending on relative ego strength is in contrast to biological views. Rather than representing polar ends of the serotonergic axis, impulsivity and compulsivity in a psychodynamic model can arise concurrently or at different times in one person depending on the balance between drives and affects and the ego mechanisms that regulate them.

The psychoanalytic metapsychological perspective may ultimately be more helpful in developing an understanding of impulsive and compulsive character traits or personality disorders such as borderline personality disorder or OCPD than in elucidating full-blown Axis I impulsive or compulsive syndromes such as pyromania or OCD. By analogy, psychodynamic views of the origins of melancholia have proven less helpful in the psychotherapy of depression than those views in which depressive affects are conceptualized according to an object relations model. Further, psychoanalytic models may be at their most informative when they examine not only traits but also the absence of trait as pathological. For example, the absence of depressive affects in appropriate intrapsychic situations can be as pathological as the presence of such affects. By extension, the absence of an appropriate capacity for impulsivity (spontaneity) is a defining feature of OCPD, whereas the absence of a normal degree of compulsivity (carefulness) is a pathological aspect of borderline personality disorder. Psychoanalytic principles remain most illuminating and clinically relevant when drawn on to address the relative balance of impulsive and compulsive traits needed for optimal functioning in love, work, and play.

# References

American Psychiatric Association: Diagnostic and Statistical Manual of Mental Disorders, 3rd Edition, Revised. Washington, DC, American Psychiatric Association, 1987

American Psychiatric Association: Diagnostic and Statistical Manual of Mental Disorders, 4th Edition. Washington, DC, American Psychiatric Association, 1994

Arlow JA, Brenner C: Psychoanalytic Concepts and the Structural Theory. New York, International Universities Press, 1964

Baer L, Jenike MA: Personality disorders in obsessive-compulsive disorder. Psychiatr Clin North Am 15:803–812, 1992

Brenner C: An Elementary Textbook of Psychoanalysis. New York, International Universities Press, 1973

Brenner C: The Mind in Conflict. Madison, CT, International Universities Press, 1982

Cloninger CR, Svrakic DM, Przybeck TR: A psychobiological model of temperament and character. Arch Gen Psychiatry 50:975–990, 1993

Deutsch H: Some forms of emotional disturbance and their relationships to schizophrenia. Psychoanal Q 11:301–321, 1942

Esman AH: Psychoanalysis and general psychiatry: obsessive-compulsive disorder as paradigm. J Am Psychoanal Assoc 37:319–336, 1989

Fairbairn WRD: An Object-Relations Theory of the Personality. New York, Basic Books, 1954

Fairbairn WRD: Synopsis of an object-relations theory of the personality. Int J Psychoanal 44:224–226, 1963

Freud S: Further remarks on the neuro-psychoses of defence (1896), in Standard Edition of the Complete Psychological Works of Sigmund Freud, Vol 3. Translated and edited by Strachey J. London, Hogarth Press, 1962, pp 157–185

Freud S: Character and anal erotism (1908), in Standard Edition of the Complete Psychological Works of Sigmund Freud, Vol 9. Translated and edited by Strachey J. London, Hogarth Press, 1959, pp 167–175

Freud S: Notes upon a case of obsessional neurosis (1909), in Standard Edition of the Complete Psychological Works of Sigmund Freud, Vol 10. Translated and edited by Strachey J. London, Hogarth Press, 1955, pp 151–318

Freud S: Remembering, repeating and working-through (further recommendations on the technique of psycho-analysis II) (1914), in Standard Edition of the Complete Psychological Works of Sigmund Freud, Vol 12. Translated and edited by Strachey J. London, Hogarth Press, 1958, pp 145–156

Freud S: Introductory lectures on psychoanalysis, Part III: General theory of the neuroses, Lecture XXIII: the paths to the formation of symptoms (1917[1916–1917]), in Standard Edition of the Complete Psychological Works of Sigmund Freud, Vol 16. Translated and edited by Strachey J. London, Hogarth Press, 1963, pp 358–377

Frosch EJ, Frosch JP, Frosch J: The impulse disorders (Chapter 25), in Psychiatry, Vol 1. Edited by Michels R, Cavenar JO Jr, Brodie HKH, et al. Philadelphia, PA, JB Lippincott, 1993

Frosch J: The relation between acting out and disorders of impulse control. Psychiatry 40:295–314, 1977

Gabbard GO: Psychodynamic psychiatry in the "Decade of the Brain." Am J Psychiatry 149:991–998, 1992

Greenberg JR, Mitchell SA: Object Relations in Psychoanalytic Theory. Cambridge, MA, Harvard University Press, 1983

Ingram DH: Compulsive personality disorder. Am J Psychoanal 42: 189–198, 1982

Joffee RT, Swinson RP, Regan JJ: Personality features of obsessive-compulsive disorder. Am J Psychiatry 145:1127–1129, 1988

Kaplan AH: Obsessive-compulsive phenomena in adult obsessionality, compulsive personality disorder and obsessive-compulsive disorder (neurosis). Psychiatric Journal of the University of Ottawa 12:214–221, 1987

Katz RJ: Neurobiology of obsessive compulsive disorder: a serotonergic basis of Freudian repression. Neurosci Biobehav Rev 15:375–381, 1991

Kernberg OF: Borderline Conditions and Pathological Narcissism. New York, Jason Aronson, 1975

Kernberg OF: Object Relations and Clinical Psychoanalysis. New York, Jason Aronson, 1976

Kernberg OF: Severe Personality Disorders: Psychotherapeutic Strategies. New Haven, CT, Yale University Press, 1984

Kernberg OF: Hysterical and histrionic personality disorders (Chapter 19), in Psychiatry, Vol 1. Edited by Michels R, Cavenar JO Jr, Brodie HKH, et al. Philadelphia, PA, JB Lippincott, 1985

Kernberg OF, Selzer MA, Koenigsberg HW, et al: Psychodynamic Psychotherapy of Borderline Patients. New York, Basic Books, 1990

Klein DF: Psychopharmacological treatment and delineation of borderline disorders, in Borderline Personality Disorders: The Concept, the Syndrome, the Patient. Edited by Hartocollis P. New York, International Universities Press, 1977, pp 365–384

Krueger DW: On compulsive shopping and spending: a psychodynamic inquiry. Am J Psychother 42:574–584, 1988

Lansky MR: The explanation of impulsive action. British Journal of Psychotherapy 6:10–25, 1989

Lidz T: Family studies and changing concepts of personality development. Can J Psychiatry 24:621–631, 1979

MacKinnon RA, Michels R: The Psychiatric Interview in Clinical Practice. Philadelphia, PA, WB Saunders, 1971

Mollinger RN: Antithesis and the obsessive-compulsive. Psychoanal Rev 67:465–477, 1980

Munich R: Transitory symptom formation in the analysis of an obsessional character. Psychoanal Study Child 41:515–536, 1986

Nagera H: Obsessional Neuroses: Developmental Psychopathology. New York, Jason Aronson, 1976

Oldham JM, Frosch WA: Compulsive personality disorder (Chapter 22), in Psychiatry, Vol 1. Edited by Michels R, Cavenar JO Jr, Brodie HKH, et al. Philadelphia, PA, JB Lippincott, 1985

Oldham JM, Clarkin J, Appelbaum A, et al: A self-report instrument for borderline personality organization, in The Borderline: Current Empirical Research. Edited by McGlashan TH. Washington, DC, American Psychiatric Press, 1985, pp 1–18

Pfohl B, Blum N: Obsessive-compulsive personality disorder: a review of available data and recommendations for DSM-IV. Journal of Personality Disorders 5:363–375, 1991

Pitman RK, Jenike MA: Normal and disordered compulsivity: evidence against a continuum. J Clin Psychiatry 50:450–452, 1989

Pollak J: Obsessive-compulsive personality: theoretical and clinical perspectives in recent research findings. Journal of Personality Disorders 1:248–262, 1987a

Pollak J: Relationship of obsessive-compulsive personality to obsessive-compulsive disorder: a review of the literature. Journal of Psychology 121:137–148, 1987b

Rado S: Obsessive behavior: so-called obsessive-compulsive neurosis, in American Handbook of Psychiatry, 2nd Edition (Arieti S, Editor-in-Chief), Vol 3: Adult Clinical Psychiatry. Edited by Arieti S, Brody EB. New York, Basic Books, 1974, pp 195–208

Reich W: Character Analysis (1933). Translated by Wolfe TP. New York, Orgone Institute Press, 1945

Rosenberg E: Anxiety and the capacity to bear it. Int J Psychoanal 30:1–12, 1949

Salzman L: The Obsessive Personality: Origins, Dynamics and Therapy. New York, Science House, 1968

Salzman L: Treatment of the Obsessive Personality. New York, Jason Aronson, 1980

Sandler J: On the concept of superego. Psychoanal Study Child 15:128–162, 1960

Sandler J, Holder A, Meers D: The ego ideal and the ideal self. Psychoanal Study Child 18:139–158, 1963

Shapiro D: Neurotic Styles. New York, Basic Books, 1965

Shapiro D: Autonomy and Rigid Character. New York, Basic Books, 1981

Stone MH: Borderline personality disorder (Chapter 17), in Psychiatry, Vol 1. Edited by Michels R, Cavenar JO Jr, Brodie HKH, et al. Philadelphia, PA, JB Lippincott, 1988

Sutherland JD: The British object relations theorists: Balint, Winnicott, Fairbairn, Guntrip. J Am Psychoanal Assoc 28:829–860, 1980

Svrakic DM, Whitehead C, Przybeck TR, et al: Differential diagnosis of personality disorders by the seven-factor model of temperament and character. Arch Gen Psychiatry 50:991–999, 1993

Thomas A, Chess S, Birch H, et al: Behavioral Individuality in Early Childhood. New York, New York University Press, 1963

Thompson JM, Baxter LR, Schwartz JM: Freud, obsessive-compulsive disorder and neurobiology. Psychoanalysis and Contemporary Thought 15:483–505, 1992

Winnicott DW: The theory of the parent-infant relationship (1960), in The Maturational Processes and the Facilitating Environment. New York, International Universities Press, 1965, pp 37–55

Winnicott DW: Ego distortion in terms of true and false self, in The Maturational Processes and the Facilitating Environment. New York, International Universities Press, 1965, pp 140–152

Wurmser L: Denial and split identity: timely issues in the psychoanalytic psychotherapy of compulsive drug users. J Subst Abuse Treat 2:89–96, 1985

Zetzel E: The so-called good hysteric. Int J Psychoanal 49:256–260, 1968

# 8

# Defense Mechanisms in Impulsive Versus Obsessive-Compulsive Disorders

J. Christopher Perry, M.P.H., M.D.

## Background

### Freud

Sigmund Freud first described defensive operations in "The Neuro-Psychoses of Defence" (S. Freud 1894/1962). He recounted case vignettes in which dramatic symptoms, usually diagnosed as

Collection of data reported in this chapter was supported by a grant from the National Institute of Mental Health (R01 MH-34123) while the author was at The Cambridge Hospital, Cambridge, Massachusetts. Chapter based on paper presented at the 145th annual meeting of the American Psychiatric Association, Washington, D.C., May 7, 1992.

hysterical phobias or obsessions, appeared to result from prohibitions against strong wishes, which themselves were kept out of awareness. In these vignettes he referred to the idea of *defense* or *repression*, terms that he used synonymously, as an intentional effort to forget incompatible ideas. Although Freud later noted that his theory of repression or defense was at the base of psychoanalysis (S. Freud 1914/1957), he never fully systematized knowledge about defenses. This task was later carried out by others, foremost of whom was his daughter, Anna Freud (1936/1937), who wrote *The Ego and the Mechanisms of Defence*, and later Fenichel (1945), who systematically presented what others had written about defenses, character, and symptom formation.

In Freud's 1894 paper he first described the defensive phenomena underlying obsessions. According to Freud, affect is separated from its relevant idea, thereby weakening the mental effect of the idea, and the affect is then reattached to other ideas that are not incompatible but are, in fact, symbolically related to the weakened idea. Later in the article, Freud used the terms isolation and displacement to describe these defensive processes. Subsequently, in "Inhibitions, Symptoms and Anxiety," Freud (1926/1959) further specified that regression, reactive alteration of the ego (i.e., reaction formation), isolation, and undoing were involved in obsessions, a point also noted by Anna Freud (1937/1936, p. 46).

## Fenichel

Fenichel (1945) pointed out similarities between those patients with obsessions and compulsions and those with impulse neuroses, or what today we would characterize as impulsive behavior:

> Perverse activities and the impulses of "psychopaths" (such as the drive to run away, cleptomania, or drug addiction) sometimes are designated as compulsion symptoms because the patients feel "compelled" to carry out their pathological action. . . . More characteristic is the difference in the way the urge is felt. The compulsion neurotic feels forced to do something that he does not *like* to do, that is, compelled to use his

volition against his own desires; the pervert feels forced to "like" something, even against his will. Guilt feelings may oppose his impulses; nevertheless[,] at the moment of his excitement he feels the impulse as ego syntonic, as a something he wants to do in the hope of achieving positive pleasure. (p. 324)

Thus, Fenichel suggests that there should be dynamic differences in the defenses underlying these two broad groups of disorders.

Although Fenichel, in his description of the dynamics of the impulse neuroses, focused on their intrapsychic symbolic meanings, his treatment of the use of these defenses was left to the interstices of his text. Nonetheless, the following defenses can reasonably be inferred in his descriptions.

*Passive aggression* is congruent with Fenichel's description of one dynamic in masochism as "hostility . . . turned against one's own ego" (Fenichel 1945, p. 360). It is also embedded alongside another description of masochism in which *help-rejecting complaining* (hypochondriasis) is clearly described:

Masochistic characters customarily derive pleasure from exhibiting their misery. "Look how miserable I am" typically stands for "Look how miserable you have made me"; the masochistic behavior has an accusing, blackmailing tone; the sadism, which has been turned against the ego in masochism, returns in the way the patients attempt to force their objects to give love or affection. (Fenichel 1945, p. 363)

Finally, as a general comment about other forms of impulsive behavior, Fenichel noted that the analyst would have to show certain modifications in treatment to help the patient deal with "the intolerance of tension and the tendency to 'act out'" (p. 386). Thus, in his description of both impulsive and self-destructive or masochistic behaviors, Fenichel described the three defenses passive aggression, help-rejecting complaining (hypochondriasis), and acting out, which I have elsewhere called the *action defenses* (Perry and Cooper 1985, 1986, 1989).

Fenichel (1945) discussed the role of defenses in only a few specific impulsive disorders. Fenichel's writings on the dynamics of eating disorders are limited. He noted that *repression* of certain conflicts is found in both anorectic (p. 176) and bulimic (pp. 176, 381) conditions. He described related phenomena of specific eating taboos, noting that such beliefs are *rationalized* or *idealized* (p. 176). Finally, he noted that anorexia may be multidetermined as a simple hysterical symptom (repression) or an ascetic *reaction formation* in a compulsion neurosis (p. 176). Overall, in Fenichel's view, the importance of repression is clear in both bulimia and anorexia, and the latter may also involve reaction formation. In the context of examining the psychodynamics of suicide, Fenichel described passive aggression: "The suicide of the depressed patient is, if examined from the standpoint of the superego, a turning of sadism against the person himself, and the thesis that nobody kills himself who had not intended to kill somebody else is proved by the depressive suicide" (p. 400).

## Kernberg

From the theoretical vantage point of object relations, Kernberg (1967), who has focused so well on severe character problems, noted that impulse neuroses are generally associated with the borderline level of personality organization. He posited that this level includes the defenses of *splitting, projective identification, denial, primitive idealization, omnipotence,* and *devaluation.* The resort to impulsive behavior generally results from the inability to tolerate ambivalent feelings toward others, stimulated by the fluid emergence of conflicting partial object representations and the reliance on the above-mentioned defenses.

# Hypotheses

In this chapter I test the following general predictions, which are based on the partial review of the theoretical literature presented in the preceding section, by examining data on an available sample of individuals with personality and affective disorders:

1. Impulsive symptoms that are more ego-syntonic will be related to action-oriented defenses that permit expression of impulses and affects without regard to the consequences (acting out, passive aggression, and help-rejecting complaining), as well as to defenses associated with borderline personality organization as described by Kernberg (hereafter designated as major and minor image-distorting defenses). The relationships will be strongest for the most self-destructive impulses.
2. Obsessive-compulsive symptoms that are ego-dystonic will be related to the neurotic-level defenses of isolation, undoing, displacement, and reaction formation, which are theoretically associated with symptom formation.
3. The special impulsive symptoms relating to food will, in terms of the defenses prevalent, lie midway between self-destructive impulsive behaviors and obsessive-compulsive symptoms in that they demonstrate associations with the neurotic-level defenses of repression and reaction formation as well as lower-level defenses such as idealization (minor image-distorting) and rationalization (disavowal).

## Methods

The data for this report are taken from my longitudinal study of borderline personality disorder (BPD). In this study we compared BPD with antisocial personality disorder, schizotypal personality disorder, and bipolar II affective disorder. The initial sample was collected in 1980–1982, with additional subjects entered in 1985–1987, including especially those with schizotypal personality disorder. All subjects were outpatients or symptomatic volunteers, and data on sample collection and diagnosis are available elsewhere (Perry 1985; Perry and Cooper 1985, 1989). In this report I focus on the relationship between defenses and specific symptoms and symptomatic behaviors rather than on diagnosis.

## Study Design

### Intake

At intake, subjects were systematically interviewed about the life-time prevalence, to date, of eight types of impulsive behaviors: suicidal thoughts, suicide attempts, wrist cutting, other self-mutilation/mortification, periods of withdrawal, binge eating, anorexia, and risk taking. Each subject was then interviewed by an independent clinician blind to all other data who conducted a dynamic interview, which was videotaped. The taped interview was subsequently rated for defenses (see below).

### Follow-Along

The subjects then entered a follow-along portion of the study, which consisted of two phases.

*Phase 1.* Between 1980 and 1983, each subject was interviewed every 3 to 6 months (median = 20.5 weeks) by research assistants. At each interview, levels of alcohol/drug abuse and antisocial symptomatology, as determined by scores on the Alcohol, Drug Abuse, and Antisocial Symptom scales from the Psychiatric Status Schedule (PSS; Spitzer et al. 1970), were obtained for the preceding month. The general level of symptoms for each subject over the whole Phase 1 follow-up period was summarized by the median score on each scale.

*Phase 2.* In 1983, a new interview format was introduced, the Longitudinal Interval Follow-Up Evaluation—Adapted for the Study of Personality (LIFE-ASP). Each subject from Phase 1 and those admitted in 1986–1987 were interviewed every 6 months. The occurrence of each behavior was recorded in a follow-along design as follows. Week-by-week ratings were available for episodes of obsessive-compulsive disorder (OCD) and for the eight impulse symptoms about which subjects had been interviewed at intake.

Each subject's course throughout Phase 2 was summarized for

each symptom by calculating the proportion of the follow-along in which the symptoms were present. Although symptom severity ratings were also available, these did not prove to change the subsequent analyses, and they are therefore omitted from this discussion for parsimony. Data from intake and follow-along on the impulsive behaviors have been previously presented (van der Kolk et al. 1991).

## Defenses

Defenses were rated from the intake videotaped interviews by use of my Defense Mechanisms Rating Scales (DMRS). The scales, rating method, and their reliability have been described in detail elsewhere (Perry 1988, 1990; Perry and Cooper 1985, 1986, 1989; Perry and Kardos 1994). Groups of three raters viewed each tape and, after making individual ratings, formed a consensus rating of 22 defenses. Scores for the eight mature defense scales were not available except for the last 31 subjects and are therefore omitted from these analyses. The ratings represented whether each defense was qualitatively absent (0), probably present (1), or definitely present (2). Defenses that were conceptually and empirically correlated were grouped into defense summary scales (median reliability intraclass R = .74), as follows:

1. *Action:* passive aggression, acting out, help-rejecting complaining
2. *Major image-distorting (borderline):* splitting of self and others' images, projective identification
3. *Disavowal:* denial, projection, rationalization; although not a disavowal defense, fantasy was also scored at this level
4. *Minor image-distorting (narcissistic):* idealization, omnipotence, devaluation
5. *Neurotic level:* a) hysterical: repression and dissociation; b) other neurotic: reaction formation and displacement
6. *Obsessional:* isolation of affect, intellectualization, undoing
7. *Mature:* affiliation, altruism, anticipation, humor, self-assertion, self-observation, sublimation, suppression

A summary scale, Overall Defensive Functioning (ODF) (for-
merly called Overall Defense Maturity), was incorporated as
follows.

Each instance of a defense rated present was weighted according to its place in the aforementioned empirically validated hierarchy from least (1) to most (6) adaptive (Perry and Cooper 1989).
The ODF score was calculated as the average weight for all the
defenses rated, and in this chapter it varies over a theoretical range
of 1 to 6 instead of 1 to 7 because of the omission of mature defenses
at the top of the hierarchy. The relative paucity of mature defenses
rated in the last 31 subjects demonstrated that the omission of this
defense level did not result in significant distortion of the ODF. To
limit the problem of multiple comparisons, subsequent data analyses used the six summary scores for the defense levels and autistic
fantasy along with the ODF only, instead of using scores for all
22 defenses.

# Results

## Impulse Histories at Intake

The prevalence of impulses in the sample at intake was high. Half
of the sample reported suicidal thoughts sometimes (i.e., more
than once or twice), half had made at least one suicide attempt,
and half had committed one act of self-cutting or other self-
mortification. Risk taking, summed across five different types of
risks (e.g., driving dangerously fast, having unprotected sex, making provocative comments that might invite attack) was common,
yielding a median of 6 (Table 8–1). Periods of complete social withdrawal or isolation and of binge eating were also found in more
than half the sample. The least common impulse problem was
periods of anorexia, defined as restrictive eating not due to depression or dieting.

**Table 8–1.**   History of self-destructive impulses in study sample at intake ($N = 109$)

| Impulse problem | Mean ± SD | Median |
|---|---|---|
| Suicidal ideation[a] | 2.2 ± 1.2 | 2.0 |
| Suicide attempts[b] | 1.4 ± 1.8 | 1.0 |
| Self-cutting[b] | 1.1 ± 1.7 | 0.0 |
| Other self-destructive behaviors[b] | 1.3 ± 2.0 | 0.0 |
| Binge eating[a] | 1.4 ± 1.5 | 0.5 |
| Anorectic periods[a] | 1.1 ± 1.3 | 0.0 |
| Periods of withdrawal[a] | 2.6 ± 1.4 | 3.0 |
| Risk taking (sum of 5 categories)[a] | 6.0 ± 4.2 | 6.0 |

[a]Five-point scale of lifetime frequency: 0 = Never; 1 = Once or twice; 2 = Sometimes; 3 = Often; 4 = Very often, almost daily.
[b]Six-point scale of raw count with truncated upper limit: 0 = 0 times; 1 = 1 time; 2 = 2 times; 3 = 3 times; 4 = 4 times; 5 = 5 or more times.

## Defenses at Intake

The defense summary scale scores for the defenses within each of the six levels of defense at intake are presented in Table 8–2. Each number represents the sum of the qualitative scores for the defenses within a level divided by the total sum of all defense scores. This figure is interpretable as the proportion of all defensive functioning attributable to the defenses in that level. For instance, the action defenses, including acting out, passive aggression, and help-rejecting complaining, account for 15.9% (.159) of all qualitative defensive functioning in this sample. The most prevalent defenses listed are the three disavowal defenses, at 20.5%. When all of the defenses below the so-called neurotic level (i.e., below displacement/reaction formation) are combined, 67.0% of the defenses identified in this sample are in levels theoretically associated with personality disorders (not shown in table; see Perry 1993). Unfortunately, mature defense scores were not available for the entire sample to complete the picture. However, as noted earlier in this chapter, data from the last 31 subjects suggest that omission of these scores results in little distortion.

**Table 8–2.**  Proportion of all defensive functioning in study sample due to each defense summary scale score ($N = 108$)

| Defense summary scale[a]              | Mean  | SD      | Median | Range       |
|---------------------------------------|-------|---------|--------|-------------|
| 6. Obsessional                        | .166  | ± .087  | .167   | .000–.428   |
| 5. Hysterical                         | .082  | ± .056  | .080   | .000–.250   |
| Displacement/reaction formation       | .080  | ± .054  | .083   | .000–.188   |
| 4. Minor image-distorting             | .146  | ± .069  | .149   | .000–.333   |
| 3. Disavowal                          | .205  | ± .064  | .200   | .056–.375   |
| Autistic fantasy                      | .024  | ± .036  | .000   | .000–.133   |
| 2. Major image-distorting             | .136  | ± .078  | .140   | .000–.357   |
| 1. Action                             | .159  | ± .075  | .151   | .000–.333   |
| Overall Defensive Functioning (1 to 6)| 3.52  | ± 0.43  | 3.52   | 2.55–4.64   |

[a]Mature defenses were only rated on the last 31 subjects admitted in 1985–1986 and are not included. The Overall Defensive Functioning scale is minimally affected because of the low prevalence of mature defenses in the sample (see text for details).

## Associations Between Impulses and Defenses

### At Intake

Associations between the most self-destructive impulses at intake and defenses, as grouped into defense summary scales, were examined (Table 8–3). *Suicidal ideation* was associated with action and major image-distorting defenses but was negatively associated with autistic fantasy and minor image-distorting defenses. *Suicide attempts* showed the same profile but with a stronger negative association with autistic fantasy and no significant association with minor image-distorting defenses. Both suicidal ideation and suicide attempts were associated with lower overall defensive functioning (as measured by ODF) than was true for the other impulses. *Self-cutting* had slightly different associations. It, too, was associated with major image-distorting defenses but showed a moderate negative association with disavowal and negative trends with minor image-distorting and displacement/reaction formation defenses.

**Table 8–3.**    Proportional defense summary scale scores and impulsive behaviors in study sample at intake ($N = 102$)

| Defense summary scale | Suicidal ideation | Suicide attempts | Self-cutting | Other self-destructive behavior |
|---|---|---|---|---|
| 7. Mature[a] | | | | |
| 6. Obsessional | −.09 | −.11 | .03 | −.01 |
| 5. Hysterical | −.04 | −.15 | .05 | .06 |
| Displacement/ reaction formation | −.10 | −.01 | −.18† | −.12 |
| 4. Minor image-distorting | −.19† | −.09 | −.18† | −.10 |
| 3. Disavowal | −.14 | −.06 | −.25** | −.03 |
| Autistic fantasy | −.16† | −.25** | −.07 | .01 |
| 2. Major image-distorting | .30** | .20* | .26** | .10 |
| 1. Action | .22* | .22* | .13 | .06 |
| Overall Defensive Functioning[a] | −.23* | −.22* | −.13 | −.05 |

[a]Mature defenses were only rated on the last 31 subjects admitted in 1985–1987 and are not included. The Overall Defensive Functioning scale is minimally affected because of the low prevalence of mature defenses in the sample (see text for details).
†$P < .10$; *$P < .05$; **$P < .01$; ***$P < .001$.

*Other self-destructive behaviors* showed no significant associations.

Associations between the other impulses at intake and defenses were also examined (Table 8–4). *Binge eating* showed only a negative association with action defenses, and *anorectic periods* were associated negatively with autistic fantasy. *Periods of withdrawal* displayed no significant associations. *Risk taking* was moderately associated with disavowal defenses and less so with minor image-distorting defenses but was negatively associated with hysterical defenses.

*Multiple regression analysis.*    Because of the multiple associations between impulses and defenses, stepwise multiple regressions were computed to determine whether different defenses contributed unique variance to each specific impulse (Table 8–5). It was found that defenses explained from 5% to 18% of the variance (median 12%) for six of the eight impulse histories assessed at intake. The results are summarized as follows:

▌ *Suicidal ideation.* Together, major image-distorting, action, and obsessional defenses predicted 18% of the variance in the frequency of suicidal ideation.

▌ *Suicide attempts.* The use of major image-distorting and action defenses, coupled with the absence of autistic fantasy, predicted 12% of the variance in the number of suicide attempts

**Table 8–4.**    Spearman correlations for defense summary scale scores and impulsive behaviors in study sample at intake ($N = 102$)

| Defense summary scale | Binge eating | Anorectic periods | Withdrawal periods | Risk taking |
|---|---|---|---|---|
| 7. Mature[a] | | | | |
| 6. Obsessional | .04 | −.08 | −.07 | −.01 |
| 5. Hysterical | .13 | .13 | .08 | −.26** |
| Displacement/ reaction formation | −.10 | −.13 | .05 | −.07 |
| 4. Minor image- distorting | .01 | −.09 | −.10 | .17† |
| 3. Disavowal | .01 | .08 | −.04 | .34*** |
| Autistic fantasy | .03 | −.20* | .04 | −.09 |
| 2. Major image- distorting | .14 | .09 | −.03 | −.15 |
| 1. Action | −.21* | .14 | .13 | .09 |
| Overall Defensive Functioning[a] | .09 | −.11 | −.05 | −.05 |

[a]Mature defenses were only rated on the last 31 subjects admitted in 1985–1986 and are not included. The Overall Defensive Functioning scale is minimally affected because of the low prevalence of mature defenses in the sample (see text for details).
†$P < .10$; *$P < .05$; **$P < .01$; ***$P < .001$.

**Table 8–5.**  Proportional defense summary scale scores as predictors of impulsive symptoms in study sample at intake: stepwise multiple regression analysis

| Symptom | Predictor | df | Beta | F | P | Cumulative $R^2$ |
|---|---|---|---|---|---|---|
| | | | | *Stepwise multiple regression* | | |
| Suicidal ideation | Major image-distorting | 3,97 | 6.17 | 9.12 | .003 | .08 |
| | Action | | 4.76 | 6.11 | .02 | .14 |
| | Obsessional | | 3.22 | 4.41 | .04 | .18 |
| Suicide attempts | Fantasy | 3,97 | −11.2 | 6.58 | .01 | .06 |
| | Major image-distorting | | 4.17 | 3.54 | .06 | .10 |
| | Action | | 3.77 | 2.59 | .11 | .12 |
| Self-cutting | Major image-distorting | 4,96 | 7.32 | 4.04 | .05 | .04 |
| | Obsessional | | 4.39 | 2.46 | .12 | .06 |
| | Action | | 5.28 | 3.06 | .08 | .09 |
| | Hysterical | | 5.16 | 2.64 | .11 | .12 |
| Other self-destructive behavior | | | | ——Not significant—— | | |
| Binge eating | Action | 1,99 | −4.82 | 5.64 | .02 | .05 |
| Anorectic periods | Fantasy | 3,97 | −6.03 | 3.91 | .05 | .04 |
| | Action | | 4.01 | 2.72 | .10 | .06 |
| | Hysterical | | 4.76 | 4.14 | .04 | .10 |
| Periods of withdrawal | | | | ——Not significant—— | | |
| Risk taking | Disavowal | 3,97 | 18.03 | 8.01 | .006 | .07 |
| | Minor image-distorting | | 12.83 | 3.54 | .06 | .11 |
| | Action | | 8.57 | 2.31 | .13 | .13 |

by history. Fantasy appears to offer a protective effect against turning anger against the self and self-representations.

I *Self-cutting.* Major image-distorting and action defenses, coupled with both obsessional and hysterical defenses, predicted 12% of the variance in the number of self-cutting episodes.

I *Other self-destructive impulses.* No variance was explained by the defenses.

I *Binge eating.* The only association found was negative: (the absence of) action defenses predicted 5% of the variance in the reported frequency of binge-eating episodes. This finding suggests that binge eating is dynamically healthier than the self-destructive impulses (suicidal ideation, suicide attempts, self-cutting), which were positively associated with action defenses.

I *Anorectic periods.* Hysterical and action defenses, coupled with the absence of autistic fantasy, predicted 10% of the variance in reported frequency of anorectic periods.

I *Periods of withdrawal.* No variance was explained by the defenses.

I *Risk taking.* Disavowal, minor image-distorting, and, to a lesser extent, action defenses were associated with an amalgam of risk-taking episodes.

**On Follow-Up**

*Phase 1 (Psychiatric Status Schedule).* Impulse symptom data, available from the PSS scales during Phase 1 follow-up for 67 subjects, have previously been reported (Perry and Cooper 1989) and are summarized here. Subjects had a range of two to seven follow-up administrations of the PSS. At intake, defenses from the lower half of the hierarchy of adaptation predicted the median scores of three impulse symptom scales on the PSS.

I *Antisocial behaviors* were predicted by the action ($r = .30$, $P < .05$), disavowal ($r = .33$, $P < .01$), and minor image-distorting ($r = .25$, $P < .05$) defenses.

I *Alcohol abuse* symptoms were predicted by the action ($r = .29$, $P < .05$) and disavowal ($r = .32$, $P < .01$) defenses.

▌ *Drug abuse* was predicted only by the action defense ($r = .33$, $P < .01$).

Neither the major image-distorting nor the obsessional defenses predicted either substance abuse or antisocial symptoms. These findings generally confirm hypothesis 1 (see section on hypotheses earlier in this chapter).

*Phase 2 (LIFE-ASP).*    Data from the LIFE-ASP follow-along interviews were available for 93 individuals. Each impulsive symptom was summarized by the proportion of total follow-along during which it was present (see data in Tables 8–6 and 8–7). The mean length of follow-along for the impulse symptoms was 159.6 ± 97.7 weeks.

▌ *Suicidal ideation.* Major image-distorting and action defenses were associated with the persistence of suicidal ideas. A negative correlation with obsessional and negative trends with disavowal and minor image-distorting defenses suggest that these defenses mitigated against persistent suicidal ideation. Higher overall defensive functioning, as measured by ODF scores, was also negatively associated with suicidal ideation.

▌ *Suicide attempts.* There was a trend for action defenses to be associated with the number of suicide attempts over follow-up.

▌ *Self-cutting.* This symptom had a profile similar to that for suicide attempts. Both the action and the hysterical defenses predicted the number of episodes of self-cutting on follow-up (trends only).

▌ Other self-destructive behaviors. No significant associations were obtained.

▌ *Binge eating.* Over the follow-along, there was an attentuation of the associations between binge eating and defenses at intake, resulting in no significant correlations.

▌ *Anorectic periods.* The association between defenses and periods of anorexia, in contrast to binge eating, increased over the follow-along. Action defenses and autistic fantasy (trend only) were positively associated with anorectic periods, whereas

**Table 8–6.** Proportional defense summary scale scores and impulsive behaviors in study sample on follow-up ($N = 93$)

| Defense summary scale | Suicidal ideation | Suicide attempts | Self-cutting | Other self-destructive behavior |
|---|---|---|---|---|
| 7. Mature[a] | | | | |
| 6. Obsessional | −.28** | −.10 | −.14 | −.05 |
| 5. Hysterical | .09 | .09 | .19† | .07 |
|    Displacement/ reaction formation | −.02 | −.07 | −.06 | −.03 |
| 4. Minor image-distorting | −.19† | −.07 | −.16 | −.05 |
| 3. Disavowal | −.20† | −.03 | −.11 | −.13 |
|    Autistic fantasy | −.08 | −.16 | −.04 | .09 |
| 2. Major image-distorting | .34*** | .09 | .09 | .05 |
| 1. Action | .20* | .17† | .18† | .11 |
| Overall Defensive Functioning[a] | −.28** | −.12 | −.14 | −.05 |

[a]Mature defenses were only rated on the last 31 subjects admitted in 1985–1986 and are not included. The Overall Defensive Functioning scale is minimally affected because of the low prevalence of mature defenses in the sample (see text for details).
†$P < .10$; *$P < .05$; **$P < .01$; ***$P < .001$.

obsessional and disavowal (trend only) defenses, along with overall defensive functioning, were negatively associated with periods of restrictive eating.

▮ *Withdrawal periods.* Defenses predicted this symptom better on follow-up than at intake. Major image-distorting and action (trend only) defenses were positively associated with periods of withdrawal, whereas obsessional defenses and overall defensive functioning were negatively associated. This pattern was similar to that for suicidal ideation.

▮ *Risk taking.* No significant associations were obtained.

**Table 8–7.** Spearman correlations for defense summary scale scores and impulsive behaviors in study sample on follow-along ($N = 93$)

| | Binge eating | Anorectic periods | Withdrawal periods | Risk taking | OC symptoms[a] |
|---|---|---|---|---|---|
| 7. Mature[b] | | | | | |
| 6. Obsessional | –.02 | –.25* | –.25* | –.17 | –.02 |
| 5. Hysterical | .10 | –.04 | .07 | .04 | –.08 |
| Displacement/ reaction formation | .00 | .14 | .02 | .01 | –.06 |
| 4. Minor image-distorting | .10 | .00 | –.13 | –.07 | .03 |
| 3. Disavowal | .00 | –.19† | –.12 | –.06 | –.16 |
| Autistic fantasy | .03 | .17† | –.01 | .04 | .10 |
| 2. Major image-distorting | .02 | .12 | .25* | .05 | .18† |
| 1. Action | –.13 | .21* | .20† | .12 | –.02 |
| Overall Defensive Functioning[b] | .07 | –.21* | –.24* | –.11 | –.11 |

*Note.* OC = obsessive-compulsive.
[a]$N = 86$.
[b]Mature defenses were only rated on the last 31 subjects admitted in 1985–1986 and are not included. The Overall Defensive Functioning scale is minimally affected because of the low prevalence of mature defenses in the sample (see text for details).
†$P < .10$; *$P < .05$.

> *Obsessive-compulsive symptoms.* Major image-distorting defenses predicted obsessive-compulsive symptoms at a trend level over the follow-along.

## Stability of Impulsive Behaviors

Each impulsive symptom at intake was most highly correlated with itself over the follow-along, as one would predict. The stability correlations were as follows ($n = 91$ unless noted otherwise): suicidal ideation ($r_s = .62$, $P < .0001$), suicide attempts ($r_s = .30$, $P < .004$), self-cutting ($r_s = .44$, $P < .0001$), binge eating ($r_s = .38$, $n = 90$, $P < .0002$), anorectic periods ($r_s = .28$, $P < .006$), periods of withdrawal ($r_s = .36$, $P < .0005$), and risk taking ($r_s = .30$, $P < .003$). The one exception was that other self-destructive behavior at intake correlated with itself over follow-along ($r_s = .23$, $P < .03$) less highly than self-cutting at intake did with other self-destructive behavior on follow-up ($r_s = .39$, $P < .0001$).

## Predictive Relationship Between Defenses and Impulsive and Obsessive-Compulsive Symptoms: Multiple Regression Analysis

The strongest test of the predictive relationship between defenses and impulsive and obsessive-compulsive symptoms examined the variance explained by defenses after controlling for the variance explained by each symptom itself assessed at intake. In a series of multiple regressions, the variable to be predicted was the proportion of time symptomatic for each symptom over follow-along. Of the predictor variables, the rating of the same symptom at intake was entered first, followed by the stepwise entry of the defense levels and fantasy using a probability cutoff of $P < .15$ for entry into the equation (Table 8–8). All nine models were significant. The impulse symptoms themselves and defenses at intake together explained between 7.4% and 33.8% (median = 17.2%) of the variance in the same symptom over follow-along.

▌ *Suicidal ideation.* Obsessional defenses negatively predicted the presence of suicidal ideation over follow-along, suggesting a protective effect. Together with suicidal ideation at intake, these defenses explained 33.8% of the total variance, the highest of all the symptoms.

▌ *Suicide attempts.* The hysterical defenses together with the past number of suicide attempts explained 15.1% of the variance in suicide attempts over the follow-along.

I  *Self-cutting.* Similar to suicidal ideation, self-cutting at intake and obsessional defenses explained 24.2% of the total variance. Obsessional defenses protected against self-cutting over follow-along.

I  *Other self-destructive behaviors.* Obsessional defenses demonstrated a weak negative effect against the continuation of these behaviors. The total variance explained was 7.4%.

I  *Binge eating.* Disavowal defenses demonstrated a weak negative prediction of the continuation of binge eating. Disavowal together with binge eating at intake explained 28.6% of the total variance.

I  *Anorectic periods.* Autistic fantasy and action and displacement/reaction formation defenses predicted continuation of anorectic periods, whereas disavowal defenses again demonstrated a weak negative effect. The total variance explained was 28.0%.

I  *Periods of withdrawal.* Obsessional defenses negatively predicted the continuation of periods of withdrawal over follow-along. Obsessional defenses together with the symptom at intake explained 17.2% of the total variance.

I  *Risk taking.* Obsessional defenses predicted a negative effect on the continuation of risk taking over follow-along. Together with the symptom at intake, obsessional defenses explained 13.7% of the total variance.

I  *Obsessive-compulsive symptoms.* The symptom variable was not available from intake, and so only defenses were included in the analyses. Major image-distorting defenses and autistic fantasy together predicted 9.3% of the variance in these symptoms over follow-along.

Striking in these analyses was that the presence of obsessional defenses at intake exerted a negative effect on the continuation of five impulse symptoms over follow-along: suicidal ideation, self-cutting, other self-destructive behaviors, periods of withdrawal, and risk taking. These defenses, the most adaptive defenses rated in this sample, minimize the experience of painful feelings and apparently exerted a protective effect on self-destructive impulses. A similar but

**Table 8–8.** Proportional defense summary scale scores as predictors of impulsive symptoms at follow-up after entering impulses at intake into the analysis

| Symptom | Predictor | df | Beta | Stepwise multiple regressions | | | Cumulative $R^2$ |
|---|---|---|---|---|---|---|---|
| | | | | F | P | $R^2$ | |
| Suicidal ideation | Suicidal ideas at intake | 2,86 | .149 | 32.12 | .0001 | .254 | .254 |
| | Obsessional | | −1.217 | 11.01 | .001 | .085 | .338 |
| Suicide attempts | Attempts at intake | 2,86 | .142 | 9.95 | .002 | .092 | .092 |
| | Hysterical | | 3.33 | 6.01 | .02 | .059 | .151 |
| Self-cutting | Self-cutting at intake | 2,86 | .390 | 25.02 | .0001 | .212 | .212 |
| | Obsessional | | −3.082 | 3.46 | .07 | .031 | .242 |
| Other self-destructive behaviors | Other self-destructive behavior at intake | 2,86 | 3.639 | 4.62 | .03 | .047 | .047 |
| | Obsessional | | −64.106 | 2.57 | .11 | .028 | .074 |
| Binge eating | Binge eating at intake | 2,86 | .068 | 31.63 | .0001 | .267 | .267 |
| | Disavowal | | −.424 | 2.33 | .13 | .020 | .286 |

|  | df |  |  |  |  |  |
|---|---|---|---|---|---|---|
| **Anorectic periods** | 5,83 |  |  |  |  |  |
| Anorectic at intake |  | .037 | 11.76 | .0009 | .091 | .091 |
| Autistic fantasy |  | 1.021 | 7.29 | .008 | .071 | .162 |
| Action |  | .455 | 5.98 | .02 | .055 | .217 |
| Displacement/ reaction formation |  | .531 | 5.05 | .03 | .044 | .262 |
| Disavowal |  | -.323 | 2.11 | .15 | .018 | .280 |
| **Periods of withdrawal** | 2,86 |  |  |  |  |  |
| Withdrawal at intake |  | .079 | 9.44 | .003 | .104 | .104 |
| Obsessional |  | -1.086 | 7.09 | .009 | .068 | .172 |
| **Risk taking** | 2,86 |  |  |  |  |  |
| Risk taking at intake |  | .015 | 10.31 | .002 | .106 | .106 |
| Obsessional |  | -.410 | 3.08 | .08 | .031 | .137 |
| **Obsessive- compulsive[a]** | 2,83 |  |  |  |  |  |
| Major image-distorting |  | 1.032 | 5.11 | .03 | .057 | .057 |
| Autistic fantasy |  | 1.644 | 3.29 | .07 | .036 | .093 |

[a] Obsessive-compulsive symptoms had not been collected at intake and therefore were not available as a predictor variable of obsessive-compulsive symptoms at follow-along.

weaker observation also holds for the disavowal defenses in both eating disorders. Individuals who deny and externalize distressing conflicts have fewer problems with eating disorders.

# Discussion

## Caveats

There are three major caveats in interpreting the results of this study. First, the sample was selected to study individuals with impulsive spectrum (borderline, antisocial) and introverted spectrum (schizotypal) personality disorders, as well as bipolar II affective disorder. The sample was not selected to represent each of the impulsive or obsessive-compulsive behaviors per se. Many of the impulsive behaviors studied co-occurred in the same individuals, thus making overlapping findings more likely and discrimination between impulse symptoms difficult. In particular, most of the individuals with obsessive-compulsive symptoms met the criteria for disorders more related to impulse problems than to anxiety disorders, resulting in a problematic confound. Together, these factors place limits on the generalizability of the results, especially in regard to the obsessive-compulsive symptoms.

Second, the selection of diagnoses also biased the defenses within the sample in the direction of the least adaptive. This bias is demonstrated by the high proportion of defenses (67%) rated below the neurotic level. This restricted range resulted in a high prevalence of lower-level defenses among those who used higher-level defenses, as demonstrated by the mean ODF score of 3.52 and the top score of 4.64. A better test of hypotheses about the differential relationship between defenses and symptoms would require a wider range of average defensive functioning, including the rating of mature defenses, omitted here.

Third, defenses were measured only qualitatively, which did not reflect the variance in how often a defense is used. Quantitative assessment would result in higher assessment reliability and greater power to detect differences based on how often individuals use each defense, not just whether they use it (Perry and Kardos 1994). For instance, this study is not able to detect whether those with obsessive-compulsive symptoms use the defenses of reaction formation, displacement, isolation, and undoing *more often* than those without these symptoms, even though both groups use them sometimes.

## Hypotheses Fully or Partially Upheld

The associations between defense levels and symptoms across the four sets of analyses are summarized in Table 8–9. Presenting the results this way highlights the patterns of associations, making it easier to relate the overall results to the hypotheses.

*Hypothesis 1.*    This hypothesis is strongly upheld. The action and major image-distorting defenses were clearly related to suicidal ideation, suicide attempts, and self-cutting in half or more of the analyses. In addition, the action defenses predicted alcohol, drug, and antisocial symptoms over Phase 1 follow-along (not shown in Table 8–9). The action defenses were also associated with periods of withdrawal and risk taking, although in fewer than half of the analyses.

*Hypothesis 2.*    This hypothesis is not upheld. The obsessional defenses (isolation, undoing, intellectualization), along with reaction formation and displacement, did not differentially predict obsessive-compulsive symptoms over follow-along. Instead, the major image-distorting defenses and autistic fantasy predicted OCD symptoms in one or both of the follow-along analyses, respectively. This unhypothesized finding is likely a direct result of the sample characteristics. Elsewhere, we reported that OCD symptoms over follow-along were associated positively with schizotypal and negatively with antisocial symptoms at intake (Perry et al. 1988). Others have reported that concurrent schizotypal symptoms are a poor

**Table 8–9.**  Summary of associations between defenses and impulsive and obsessive-compulsive (OC) symptoms in the four analyses of the study sample

| Defense level | 1 Suicidal ideation | | | | 2 Suicide attempt | | | | 3 Self-cutting | | | | 4 Other self-destructive behavior | | | | 5 Binge eating | | | | 6 Periods of anorexia | | | | 7 Periods of withdrawal | | | | 8 Risk taking | | | | 9 OC symptoms[a] | | | |
|---|---|---|---|---|---|---|---|---|---|---|---|---|---|---|---|---|---|---|---|---|---|---|---|---|---|---|---|---|---|---|---|---|---|---|---|---|
| | 1 | 2 | 3 | 4 | 1 | 2 | 3 | 4 | 1 | 2 | 3 | 4 | 1 | 2 | 3 | 4 | 1 | 2 | 3 | 4 | 1 | 2 | 3 | 4 | 1 | 2 | 3 | 4 | 1 | 2 | 3 | 4 | 1 | 2 | 3 | 4 |
| Obsessional | + | | − | − | | | | | | | + | − | | | | − | | | | | − | | | | − | − | | | | | | − | − | − | − | |
| Hysterical | | | | | | | + | | | | + | + | | | | | | | | | | + | | | | | | | | − | | | | | | |
| Displacement/ reaction formation | | | | | | | | | | | − | | | | | | | | | | | | | | | | | | | | | | | | | |
| Minor image-distorting | | − | − | | | | | | | | − | | | | | | | | | | | | + | | + | + | | | | | | | | | | |
| Disavowal | − | | | | | | | | | | − | | | | | | | | | − | | − | − | | | | | | + | + | | | | | | |
| Autistic fantasy | − | | | | − | − | | | | | | | | | | | | | | | − | − | + | + | | | | | | | | | | | | + |
| Major image-distorting | + | + | + | | | + | + | + | | | + | + | | | | | | | | | | + | + | + | | | + | | | | + | | | | + | + |
| Action | + | + | + | | + | + | + | + | | | + | + | | | | | | | − | − | | + | + | + | | | + | | | | | | | | + | + |

*Note.*  Each defense is given a plus (+) or minus (−) to represent the direction of association if it demonstrated a significant (or trend) association with each impulse or symptom for any of the four sets of analyses. The four analyses are denoted by the columns labeled 1 through 4, designating the 1) intake correlational analyses, 2) intake regression analyses, 3) follow-up correlational analyses, and 4) follow-up regression analyses.
[a]Data for analyses 1 and 2 were not available.

prognostic factor for medication treatment response of OCD symptoms, although most patients with OCD do not have schizotypal personality disorder (Jenike et al. 1986a, 1986b), and only half have personality disorders in general (Baer and Jenike 1992). In our sample, a high proportion of all of the obsessive-compulsive symptoms occurred in individuals with personality disorders, including schizotypal symptoms, which is not representative of the general population of OCD patients. In this particular subset of individuals with obsessive-compulsive symptoms, major image-distorting defenses and autistic fantasy were associated with obsessive-compulsive symptoms.

*Hypothesis 3.*    This hypothesis—that eating disorders would demonstrate relationships with both lower-level and neurotic-level defenses—was upheld for anorexia but not bulimia. Periods of anorexia were clearly associated with lower defensive functioning than was binge eating, indicating that anorectic symptoms are more seriously maladaptive from a dynamic point of view. Anorexia was strongly associated with the action defenses and somewhat less so with the hysterical defenses and reaction formation/displacement, as Fenichel suggested. In contrast, binge eating showed only negative relationships to defenses. This finding suggests that in a largely personality disorder sample, action defenses, and to a lesser degree disavowal defenses, protect against binge eating. The hypothesis regarding binge eating was not upheld. Future studies should study a wider range of individuals who binge-eat, including those without personality disorders.

# Defenses and the Formation and Continuation of Symptoms

■ Case Example

A 24-year-old woman presented with major depression, dysthymia, and bulimia after a history of anorexia nervosa at age 15. She glowingly described having had a very loving positive relationship with her deceased father (idealization). Two older siblings were teasing and verbally abusive toward her, while one of them, an older brother, was frankly physically abusive. When aware of such abuse, the patient's mother was dismissive of such problems, refusing to believe the patient or telling her to deal with it herself. Her mother was otherwise emotionally neglectful, so the patient learned to keep distress to herself, believing that she was generally inadequate (self-devaluation). At age 7, the patient was sexually molested when visiting away from home. She never told anyone, figuring she would not be believed. Then dysthymia began.

Shy and mildly overweight at age 15, the patient developed anorexia characterized by intense concern with her appearance, which she incorrectly attributed as the reason why she felt so self-conscious around her peers (displacement, self-devaluation, rationalization). She focused on diet, weight, and exercise (displacement) and lost 32% of her body weight. Her father beame ill, but her mother kept the seriousness of his condition secret. When her father died, the patient was enraged at her mother, locking herself in the bathroom for half a day, and later even hitting her father's physician for contributing to hiding the truth from her (acting out). Interestingly, after 7 months' cessation, her menses returned within the week, although her anorexia worsened during mourning. Later, she was hospitalized and began to improve. Subsequently, she developed her first major depressive episode and began to exhibit bulimia rather than anorexia. She maintained the bulimia until the present. She sought therapy after getting increasingly depressed following an anniversary of her father's death.

In psychotherapy as an adult, she still idealized her father, while usually describing her mother in wholly negative terms (splitting of others' images). She did not want to discuss the sexual molestation for fear it would be upsetting (repression), but noted a continuing wish that the perpetrator would get psychological help (displacement, reaction formation). Regarding her anorexia, she was sure the return of her menses immediately following her father's death meant something, although she could not say what (repression). She remembered telling her friends that she needed to be strong for everyone else during the mourning period (reaction formation, displacement) rather than talk for herself (rationalization). Although keeping up a good front (denial), she made seven suicide attempts, from ages 17 to 24, some in which she used highly lethal means (passive aggression, acting out). At the time of interview, she met the criteria for borderline and avoidant personality disorders with self-defeating traits.

This case illustrates the complexities of the relationship between defenses and symptoms, neither of which are static. Patients use different defenses for different stressors, and comorbidity further complicates the relationship. The anorectic episode has clear signs of conflicts around caretaking adequacy, abuse, self-image, and forbidden love and sexuality, all further complicated by the idealized father's death. Repression, reaction formation, displacement, rationalization, self-devaluation, and passive aggression moved the focus from the patient's real needs, relationships, and feelings to the false focus provided by the anorectic symptoms. With the loss of the father, the patient's reliance on the action defenses (acting out, passive aggression) and splitting increased, fueling the dysthymia, major depressive episodes, and multiple suicide attempts. To disentangle the multiple relationships between defenses and symptoms would require a more quantitative appreciation of the defenses the patient used at the time of both onset or improvement in one set of symptoms and of how the defenses may have shifted (e.g., less reliance on reaction formation) when, for instance, the anorexia shifted to bulimia and major depression. Although the quantitative and repeated observations necessary to complete this picture are lacking, the following summarizes what role defenses played with each symptom in this sample.

*Suicidal ideation and attempts.*    Major image-distorting and action defenses work together to handle conflicts over anger and disappointment about unmet wishes. When anger is split off and misdirected away from its external target (splitting of other-images), negative self-images are reinforced (splitting of self-images) and anger is turned against the self (passive aggression). Help-rejecting complaining expresses the wish for help while disguising covert feelings of reproach toward significant others who are perceived as neglectful, uncaring, or hurtful. As the individual feels increasingly powerless to negotiate help or to attain significant relief, suicidal ideas may appear.

These same defenses also put the individual at risk for making suicide attempts, especially whenever conflicts over separation/abandonment are triggered (Perry 1989). Some suicide attempts in the sample under study may also have been facilitated by the repression of memories related to early trauma and neglect (van der Kolk et al. 1991), resulting in the occasional reemergence of associated painful affective states. When these painful affective states are combined with anger over currently perceived neglect, abandonment, and/or retraumatizing experiences, the individual may feel overwhelmed, as during an original traumatic experience. The resulting anger may be explosively discharged in self-destructive action (acting out) to escape a sense of helpless rage and suffering, while symbolically punishing others.

Interestingly, several lower- to mid-level defenses appear to mitigate the effects of the action and major image-distorting defenses. Autistic fantasy—the ability to gain satisfaction from a daydream that magically, if only temporarily, solves a conflict—appears to offer some protective effects, more so on suicide attempts. Similarly, disavowal (e.g., denial) and minor image-distorting defenses (e.g., omnipotence) may protect somewhat against the sense of powerlessness that fuels suicidal ideation. This finding is consistent with the previous report in this sample that the minor image-distorting defenses also protected against recurrences of acute major depression (Perry 1988).

One implication clearly emerges from the above. Clinicians treating suicidal individuals should focus on diminishing the patient's reliance on the defenses of splitting, passive aggression, help-rejecting complaining, and acting out in favor of other defenses. Some authors have described techniques to facilitate this process (Perry and Cooper 1987; Vaillant 1992). Findings from this study suggest that fantasy, denial, projection, rationalization, omnipotence, idealization, and devaluation, as well as the obviously healthier obsessional defenses, may be temporarily useful compromises for handling conflicts and stress. If these defenses are in the patient's repertoire, the clinician should support, not confront, their use during periods of suicide risk.

*Self-cutting.*    Major image-distorting and action defenses coupled with hysterical defenses were associated with self-cutting in half the analyses. Although this profile is similar to that for suicide attempts, the more consistent presence of hysterical defenses suggests that self-cutting may be more strongly associated with repressed traumatic memories. When current experiences are similar to traumatic memories, the subject may symbolically reenact the trauma, releasing reemergent feelings in a dissociated state. When the subject perceives a current person as abusive, neglectful, or abandoning, the subject reenacts an earlier scenario, playing the roles of both passive victim and perpetrator. The cutting releases the tension of conflicting fear, rage, wishes to be taken care of, and guilt. This is consistent with the previous report in this sample that childhood trauma, neglect, and separations, coupled with dissociative symptoms (not the defense) at intake, predicted cutting at intake or over follow-along (van der Kolk et al. 1991).

Again, certain defenses may offer some protection against self-cutting, including the use of disavowal, minor image-distorting defenses, and reaction formation/displacement, as well as obsessional defenses. These defenses handle strong affects, impulses, and prohibitions without directing them toward the self. Instead, they disavow, distort, redirect, or minimize the stressors and feelings triggering the conflicts. Again, the clinician should not disturb these mid-level defenses while working to diminish the reliance on action and major image-distorting defenses. Furthermore, repressed traumas and symbolically relevant events leading to dissociation need to be kept in focus, whenever salient. After first making the patient feel safe, the therapist should validate the real and symbolic traumas before negotiating limits to self-destructiveness with the patient.

*Other self-destructive impulses.*   This group of self-destructive behaviors appeared to be too heterogeneous to demonstrate anything other than a general negative relationship with obsessional defenses. It is likely that a nonspecific effect of obsessional defenses is to protect against these as well as other impulsive symptoms.

*Binge eating.*   The only associations between this symptom and defenses were negative: (the absence of) action defenses and, to a lesser extent, the disavowal defenses. This finding suggests that in this sample, binge eating was a dynamically healthier symptom than the other self-destructive impulses, including anorexia. However, this sample did not include a sufficient proportion of individuals without personality disorders who binge-eat. A less restricted sample should offer a better test of the defenses associated with binge eating.

*Anorectic periods.*   Periods of restrictive eating appear to result from both neurotic-level (e.g., repression, reaction formation) and action-level defenses. This suggests that clinicians need to have two different foci in treatment. One is to link the overt symptom with affects and impulses directed against the self instead of toward the object for which they are relevant. The second is to bring to light the repressed conflicts that promote the misdirection of affects and motives, or substitution of the affects or motives with their opposites.

   Disavowal of stress and conflict appears to play a mildly protective role, forestalling the emergence of the anorectic symptom. The role of autistic fantasy is somewhat puzzling, with a difference having been observed between intake (protective) and over the follow-along (facilitative).

*Periods of withdrawal.*   This passive impulse to retreat from the interpersonal field is a symptom that results in days lost from work, school, or social activities, and may result in job loss. Defenses did not demonstrate much relation to withdrawal until the follow-along period, when withdrawal appeared to have a profile of defenses paralleling that for suicidal ideation. This finding suggests that the symptom has a self-destructive intent, albeit expressed in passive avoidance. This suggests that the clinician should focus on mitigating the use of the action and major image-distorting level defenses rather than viewing withdrawal as if it were generated as a neurotic-level avoidance symptom. Again, the presence of obsessional defenses, which minimize the experience of troubling affects, protects against impulsive withdrawal.

*Risk taking.*    Disavowal, minor image-distorting defenses, and, to a lesser extent, action defenses were associated with an amalgam of risk-taking episodes. Disavowal implies the denial of a clear recognition of whatever precipitates taking risks, along with rationalization or projection of the motives. Minor image-distorting defenses artificially inflate the self's sense of invulnerability (omnipotence) or devalue the potential consequences of the risk (devaluation). The presence of action defenses suggests that risk taking is often the result of an inability to tolerate distressing affects such as anger or disappointment or to delay gratification by considering its consequences. This same pattern of defenses is particularly found in antisocial individuals (Perry and Cooper 1986). This pattern of defenses attenuated over the follow-along in the sample under study, as did risk taking itself, which may somewhat explain the lack of such findings over follow-along.

*Obsessive-compulsive symptoms.*    Ratings of these symptoms were not available at intake, whereas they were over follow-along. These symptoms were most associated with major image-distorting defenses and autistic fantasy. This finding probably reflects that the sample was not selected for OCD, which appears only as a comorbid disorder. Among samples restricted to personality disorders, major image-distorting defenses and autistic fantasy appear to differentiate the individuals with obsessive-compulsive symptoms. Unacceptable wishes toward the self or others may be split off and subsequently return as symbolically related obsessions and compulsions, via reaction formation (turning into their opposite) and displacement (attributed to a less-threatening object). It is also possible that in individuals who temporarily resolve conflicts through autistic fantasy, ego-syntonic ruminations and ego-dystonic obsessions are more blurred than in others. Unfortunately, a restricted sample high in comorbidity limited the examination of OCD in this sample, making a type II error likely. The following case illustrates this problem of confounding.

■ Case Example

A 26-year-old single graduate student sought psychotherapy because "my symptoms dominate my life." He recalls having been embarrassingly shy as a child and socially inhibited by a speech articulation problem. The subject blamed his mother for not recognizing the seriousness of his problems, being overinvolved, encouraging dependency, and spoiling him on the one hand, while being emotionally neglectful on the other. His father, according to the patient, was irritable, miserly, and tyrannical, given to fits of rage at times, although occasionally solicitous of the family.

The patient began having compulsive rituals as a child. When he was 9 years old, his parents had a falling out and stopped sleeping in the same room; the father moved into the brother's room, and the patient moved into his mother's room and slept in her bed. This arrangement continued until high school. His mother developed alcoholism.

In high school he began believing that he was homosexual, but in college, when he decided that he was transsexual, he had a breakdown and was hospitalized. He never had a sexual experience, claiming not to want one, but reports having many fantasies that are homosexual or in which he envisions himself being a woman having sex with a man (autistic fantasy). Since high school, the patient has not been able to think about having a real relationship because "it makes me blush with homosexual panic" (repression, dissociation). He has an intense dread that others will see him blush when anything to do with homosexuality or any word beginning with the prefix *homo-*, such as homogeneous, is mentioned (displacement). At other times he has a dread of screaming out his thoughts, such as "I'm a homosexual" (reaction formation). He has many obsessive-compulsive rituals, including hand washing for fear of germs; walking and retracing his steps for fear of missing something; checking light switches; turning over pieces of paper on the ground, obsessed with knowing what is written on them; and making magical bets. He has a very cluttered room; keeps many notes, which he cannot throw out; and studies all of the time, despite having trouble concentrating. The subject said, "I'm not sure I'd describe myself as a person at all. I'm a diseased and disordered collection of various obsessions and compulsions" (splitting of self images).

In treatment he often made abstract statements that he then qualified or retracted—for example, "One feels oneself so completely abnormal, it sets off a desperate search for normalcy of some sort [intellectualization]. Grades have always been easy, not easy, [undoing] but one way of my doing that." Regarding treatment, he said, "I crave psychiatric attention in any form [displacement]," and stated that his goal in life was to develop a facade of normality for the benefit of the outside world, despite believing that there is no real hope for him to become human (splitting of self images). Currently, the subject finds solace in attending religious services and being on the fringe of a religious support group of gay and lesbian individuals, although he is afraid to socialize with those he meets.

In treatment once, his doctor called him a dramatic person, and the patient "punished him by stopping talking to him [passive-aggression]. I would insist that I didn't have feelings [denial] and he would argue with me, so I got worse [help-rejecting complaining]."

This case illustrates the unique problems of OCD in an individual with multiple other disorders: Axis I major depressive disorder, dysthymia, and gender identity disorder; Axis II schizoid, schizotypal, and avoidant personality disorders with borderline and compulsive traits. His most prominent defenses included those associated with the personality disorders (action and major image-distorting defenses) in addition to those associated with OCD (reaction formation, displacement, undoing). Repression and dissociation appeared to be associated with his fear of his own sexuality and sexual relationships in general, as well as his gender identity disorder. Treatment proceeded slowly but well by the therapist's taking a very supportive approach, helping to find substitutes for the patient's least mature defenses, while supporting the use of neurotic-level defenses. Multiple medications were of limited value for the patient's symptoms.

## Conclusions

Defenses make important contributions to our understanding of impulsive symptoms. In the early clinical literature, there are significant observations about self-destructive impulses that the research summarized in this chapter upholds. Defenses low on the hierarchy of adaptation and the Overall Defensive Functioning scale clearly differentiated the most self-destructive defenses, such as recurrent suicidal ideation, suicide attempts, and self-cutting. In contrast, obsessional defenses clearly showed a protective role in this sample of highly impulsive individuals. Other defenses facilitated or protected against certain impulses, depending on the function of the defense. The results suggest that a focus on defenses should be a centerpiece of the clinician's approach when treating the highly impulsive self-destructive individual.

## References

Baer L, Jenike MA: Personality disorders in obsessive-compulsive disorder. Psychiatr Clin North Am 15:803–812, 1992

Fenichel O: The Psychoanalytic Theory of Neurosis. New York, WW Norton, 1945

Freud A: The Ego and the Mechanisms of Defence (1936). London, Hogarth Press, 1937

Freud S: The neuro-psychoses of defence (1894), in Standard Edition of the Complete Psychological Works of Sigmund Freud, Vol 3. Translated and edited by Strachey J. London, Hogarth Press, 1962, pp 41–68

Freud S: History of the psycho-analytic movement (1914), in Standard Edition of the Complete Psychological Works of Sigmund Freud, Vol 14. Translated and edited by Strachey J. London, Hogarth Press, 1957, pp 7–66

Freud S: Inhibitions, symptoms and anxiety (1926), in Standard Edition of the Complete Psychological Works of Sigmund Freud, Vol 20. Translated and edited by Strachey J. London, Hogarth Press, 1959, pp 75–175

Jenike MA, Baer L, Minichiello WE, et al: Coexistent obsessive-compulsive disorder and schizotypal personality disorder: a poor prognostic indicator. Arch Gen Psychiatry 43:296, 1986a

Jenike MA, Baer L, Minichiello WE, et al: Concomitant obsessive-compulsive disorder and schizotypal personality disorder. Am J Psychiatry 143:530–532, 1986b

Kernberg OF: Borderline personality organization. J Am Psychoanal Assoc 15:641–685, 1967

Perry JC: Depression in borderline personality disorder: lifetime prevalence and longitudinal course of symptoms. Am J Psychiatry 142:15–21, 1985

Perry JC: A prospective study of life stress, defenses, psychotic symptoms and depression in borderline and antisocial personality disorders and bipolar type II affective disorder. Journal of Personality Disorders 2:49–59, 1988

Perry JC: Personality disorders, suicide, and self-destructive behavior, in Suicide Understanding and Responding: Harvard Medical School Perspectives. Edited by Jacobs D, Brown H. New York, International Universities Press, 1989, pp 157–170

Perry JC: Psychological defense mechanisms in the study of affective and anxiety disorders, in Comorbidity in Anxiety and Mood Disorders. Edited by Maser J, Cloninger CR. Washington, DC, American Psychiatric Press, 1990, pp 545–562

Perry JC: The study of defense mechanisms and their effects, in Psychodynamic Treatment Research: A Guide for Clinical Practice. Edited by Miller N, Luborsky L, Barber J, et al. New York, Basic Books, 1993, pp 276–308

Perry JC, Cooper SH: Psychodynamics, symptoms, and outcome in borderline and antisocial personality disorders and bipolar type II affective disorder, in The Borderline: Current Empirical Research. Edited by McGlashan TH. Washington, DC, American Psychiatric Press, 1985, pp 21–41

Perry JC, Cooper SH: A preliminary report on defenses and conflicts associated with borderline personality disorder. J Am Psychoanal Assoc 34:865–895, 1986

Perry JC, Cooper SH: Empirical studies of psychological defense mechanisms (Chapter 30), in Psychiatry, Vol I. Edited by Michels R, Cavenar JO Jr, Brodie HKH, et al. New York, JB Lippincott, 1987

Perry JC, Cooper SH: An empirical study of defense mechanisms, I: clinical interview and life vignette ratings. Arch Gen Psychiatry 46:444–452, 1989

Perry JC, Kardos ME: A review of research using the Defense Mechanism Rating Scales, in Ego Defenses: Theory and Practice. Edited by Conte H, Plutchik R. New York, Wiley, 1994, pp 283–299

Perry JC, Lavori P, Hoke L, et al: The natural history of anxiety and affective disorders in three personality disorders. Paper presented at the 19th annual meeting of the Society for Psychotherapy Research, Santa Fe, NM, June 17, 1988

Spitzer RL, Endicott J, Fleiss J: The Psychiatric Status Schedule: a technique of evaluating psychopathology and impairment in role functioning. Arch Gen Psychiatry 23:41–55, 1970

Vaillant GE: The beginning of wisdom is never calling a patient a borderline; or, the clinical management of immature defenses in the treatment of individuals with personality disorders. Journal of Psychotherapy Practice and Research 1:117–134, 1992

van der Kolk BA, Perry JC, Herman JL: Childhood origins of self-destructive behavior. Am J Psychiatry 148:1665–1671, 1991

# 9

# Psychotherapy With Impulsive and Compulsive Patients

## Michael H. Stone, M.D.

I n the last decade great strides have been made in the pharmacology of impulsive and compulsive disorders. "Beta-blocking" agents such as atenolol and mood-regulating medications such as lithium, valproic acid, and carbamazepine have helped control many impulsive disorders; the serotonergic antidepressants have brought relief to many patients with obsessive-compulsive disorder (OCD). Despite these welcome advances, there is still a role for psychotherapy in many of these conditions. The domain of psychotherapy itself has been expanded and modified, the better to provide treatment for patients with this important group of disorders. Up to the last generation, for example, dynamic (or "psychoanalytically oriented") psychotherapy was relied on almost exclusively. The often disappointing results of the latter spurred interest in other techniques, such as the behavioral (including *ex-*

*posure*) methods pioneered by I. M. Marks and colleagues (1975).

As for the total spectrum of conditions that fall under the dual heading *impulsive* and *compulsive* and the patients with these conditions, a greater variety of disorders and a greater number of patients would be included than might be suggested by these two terms. DSM-IV (American Psychiatric Association 1994) lists five "impulsive" disorders (intermittent explosive disorder, kleptomania, pyromania, pathological gambling, and trichotillomania), while acknowledging the existence of other, presumably less common, disorders by use of the label "not otherwise specified." These disorders are referred to in DSM-IV as *impulse-control disorders not elsewhere classified*. Obsessive-compulsive disorder is not further broken down into subtypes in the manual.

But if we take a larger and more dimensional (rather than purely category-based) approach to the whole range of psychiatric conditions, we would have to recognize that *impulsivity* can often be severe, even when it does not take one of the forms outlined above, and that impulsive and compulsive elements are often commingled in the same patient, whose condition, therefore, could not easily be diagnosed under just one rubric or the other. In addition, a complete classification of these disorders should probably include certain entities encountered primarily in forensic rather than in general psychiatry and that lie admittedly outside the realm of treatable conditions. Serial sexual homicide, for example, once the entity becomes manifest through the first murder, becomes untreatable (Stone 1994). Even here, however, the clinician will occasionally encounter a patient who, having as yet harmed no one, shows many of the signs and symptoms associated with serial killing but may still be amenable to therapy. An example of such a patient is given later in this chapter.

In this chapter I pay attention to both the categorical and the dimensional, to both the relatively "pure" and mixed disorders, within the impulsive-compulsive domain. It seems fair to say at the outset that, in general, patients with disorders characterized by compulsivity are more apt to derive benefit from verbal psychotherapy than are those with disorders characterized by impulsivity. There are two interrelated reasons why this is so. First, persons who are predominantly impulsive usually have an *external* locus of control and utilize mostly *alloplastic* coping mechanisms, whereas compulsive persons as a rule have an *internal* locus of control and rely on *autoplastic* defenses. Second, those who try to change the environment (i.e., mostly utilize alloplastic coping mechanisms) rather than themselves, and who are controlled more by shame (via external sources) than by guilt, tend to externalize the origins of their difficulties in living (blaming the "other guy"), remaining themselves "faultless" (in their own view) and thus without much motivation for change. In contrast, compulsive persons are more likely to accept responsibility for their problems, perhaps even to an exaggerated and unwarranted degree, and tend as a consequence to accept "patienthood" more readily, either seeking treatment (including psychotherapy) spontaneously or at least submitting to the need for treatment with less complaint, if such need is suggested by a spouse, relative, or friend.

Although the contemporary approach to the disorders under question is often one of *combined* pharmacotherapy and psychotherapy, in actual clinical practice (as opposed to what is recommended in textbooks or in articles based on rigorously controlled patient samples), psychotherapy may end up the mainstay of treatment in certain cases, even those in which a favorable response might have been elicited. This may be because the patient either tolerates poorly all the "appropriate" drugs or, for idiosyncratic reasons, refuses to consider any medications. In these instances, the indications for psychotherapy are indeed compelling, albeit along lines that are more personal than scientific.

## Clinical Illustrations

The following clinical material is organized according to a *spectrum*: at one extreme, the vignettes concern patients who are extremely impulsive, with little or no admixture of compulsivity, and at the other, patients who exemplify "pure" OCD with no impulsive manifestations. Along the way, we will confront a variety of "mixed" types, shading from the mostly impulsive to the mostly compulsive. In some cases, the psychopathology is encompassed neatly within the DSM definitions of impulse-control disorders; in others, the clinical situation partakes of several categories and, diagnostically, defies simple categorization.

There is another point to clarify regarding category-based diagnosis. DSM-IV definitions of two "impulse-control disorders"— pyromania and kleptomania—mention as an exclusionary item the committing of these acts for reasons of anger or vengeance. Occasionally, one will encounter persons exhibiting these disorders in whom *consciously felt* emotions of this kind are not discernible. But it would be rare to work for any length of time psychotherapeutically with kleptomanic or pyromanic patients without discovering, not so far beneath the surface, enormous pools of vengeful feelings and rage. Thus, the relevance of this exclusionary item will depend on the degree to which the clinician is evaluating the impulsive patient vis-à-vis surface versus underlying psychodynamic considerations.

In the following clinical vignettes, names and identifying details have been changed to safeguard confidentiality.

## Predominantly Impulsive Disorders

Joseph, a single man in his late 20s, came for therapy at the urging of his father. His adolescence had been chaotic, made worse by alcohol abuse, which ceased only with Joseph's enrollment in Alcoholics Anonymous (AA) at age 23. He has maintained abstinence for the past 4 years. His "drinking decade" was characterized by dangerous escapades, wasteful "jet-setting" that exhausted a large inheritance, several car crashes, and an explosive episode in which he became enraged during a party, bludgeoning to death a woman who refused his advances. Curiously, the case never came to court. When I began working with him, he was still impulsive but no longer given to rage outbursts. His facade was bland. Impulsivity was now confined to such matters as hopping across country or continents on the spur of the moment for a "party," moving from one affair to the next, one job to the next, on a whim and with no fixed goal, or charging expensive outfits—which he then never wore—to his father's account. Coming to his twice-weekly sessions was the only thing he did with any regularity—at first that is, because after a few months there began to be many last-minute absences without notice, when he suddenly decided to ski in the Rockies or spend the weekend in Europe. Therapy, what there was of it, was purely supportive; my efforts were directed toward getting him settled in a job he could stay at and in a relationship that might last. Thanks to his surface affability, he was able to get a sales position with an investment house, but his stay there was short-lived because he brought in no business. Yet he spoke of making "million-dollar deals," which had no basis in fact. I only found out the truth after speaking with his relatives.

After 1½ years, Joseph stopped treatment altogether. In following up the case 4 years later, I learned that he had married a woman who was much more "solid" than he and who was seemingly unaware of his questionable past. He had been given a sinecure by someone in his family, which gave him at least the appearance of stability. Joseph's having married and obtained a job, plus his having become less impulsive, meant that he had in effect "settled down." How much to attribute to therapy and how much to growing older (and making an unexpectedly good marriage) is an open question.

❖

Terry, a married 30-year-old woman with two small children, sought therapy because of a deteriorating marital situation; having learned of her husband's infidelity, she grew depressed and, at times, suicidal. She took to having brief affairs herself, meeting men in bars in a different city and using a different name. She began to abuse alcohol, though this occurred only during the week before her period. Alcohol brought out a Jekyll and Hyde aspect to her personality: after even two drinks, she became spiteful and rageful, much in contrast to her usual shy demeanor. She went on a number of buying sprees, racking up huge bills for clothing and jewelry. Besides these impulsive actions (which also included breaking dishes during fits of pique at home), there was also compulsive behavior, which consisted of Terry's biting her fingernails almost continuously and of her primping before the mirror for 2 or 3 hours till each hair was "just so," before she could venture out of the house. Diagnostically, the patient's condition met all of the "criteria" for borderline personality disorder.

Treatment consisted at first of three sessions a week of a partly supportive/limit-setting, partly exploratory psychotherapy. Her depression lifted following a course of antidepressant medication. The episodic alcohol abuse was difficult to contain, because she refused to return to AA after the first meeting and refused to stay on Antabuse for more than a few days. Small doses of a neuroleptic (thioridazine) the week before her menses decreased the irritability.

Psychotherapy lasted 2½ years. The main theme centered around the sexual molestation experienced at the hands of her father, which had led to the divorce of her parents when she was 16, and to the interruption of her schooling. A pattern of alternating dependency on and distrust of men developed, which expressed itself through extremes of jealousy, periods of promiscuity, and choosing men with whom she could repeat the drama of use and misuse that began with her father. She tended to become frantic when alone, a situation aggravated by the absence of sustaining friendships or avocational pursuits. As part of the supportive component of her treatment, she was encouraged to enroll in art courses, because she had a distinct artistic flair. Over time, she became adept as a decorator and sculptor. These abilities helped combat the anxiety mobilized by her eventual divorce. At follow-up, 14 years later, she had remarried, divorced a second time, and was now living with a man in a more tranquil relationship. She was less jealous, had rarely touched alcohol in recent years, and supplemented the family income through occasional decorating commissions.

## Intermittent Explosive Disorder

Beatrice was referred, along with her husband, for marital therapy, by a colleague who was concerned that her tempestuousness would adversely affect both her marriage and her children. She was 35 when I first saw the couple. There were two small children by this marriage and a daughter of 12 by the husband's first marriage. Beatrice worked part-time as an editor for a magazine.

Beatrice's early years had been marred by gratuitous and severe physical abuse by her father. There were many histrionic elements in her personality—she dressed seductively, for example, wearing clothes more appropriate for a girl in her teens, and her language was dramatic and her gestures flamboyant—yet these qualities seemed only a thin camouflage for her hostility. It took very little to trigger outbursts of rage and combativeness. Three months after I began working with Beatrice and her husband, for example, it chanced that her stepdaughter had to switch her usual visiting day. Beatrice found the slightest change in plans extremely disconcerting. Shortly after the visits began, Beatrice took offense at something trivial and (in a kind of trichotillomania by proxy) pulled out a large swatch of her stepdaughter's hair. The girl ran out of the house, vowing never to return. When the couple recounted this episode in their next session, I tried to point out the destructiveness of Beatrice's ragefulness, which could not help but polarize the family and alienate her husband, on whom she was, nevertheless, quite dependent. She immediately took umbrage at my remark, cursed at me for suggesting she had a problem with anger, and stormed out of the office. She not only quit treatment, but also, for a period of several months, abandoned her husband and her own two children. As I later learned from the referring colleague, she had had a series of brief affairs, finally returning home, in a mood no less feisty and to a marriage no less turbulent than before.

## Trichotillomania and Borderline Personality Disorder

Emily, a 19-year-old woman, had been admitted because of self-mutilation to a hospital unit where I was an attending psychiatrist. She had come from a family where several members had one or another form of manic-depressive illness. Her father had been moody and volatile, sometimes showering her with attention and gifts as his "favorite," and sometimes abusing her physically without provocation. In one such instance, he twisted one of her fingers so far back as to break it.

Throughout the year before her hospitalization, Emily had become progressively more impulsive, irascible, and self-mutilative. Her arms showed "tracks" from many wrist cuttings. Even more noticeable was that she had pulled out sections of her hair with such regularity as to render herself nearly bald. To conceal this self-induced deformity, she wore a wig.

While on the unit, Emily seemed always to be looking for a fight, and she often came to blows with other patients and even with the nursing staff. Her treatment consisted mainly of thrice-weekly exploratory psychotherapy plus an antidepressant (imipramine). This medication had no effect. The serotonergic drugs were not yet available (her stay on the unit was in the early 1970s). She was not a good candidate for exploratory therapy: she was little motivated and remained much too action oriented. Supportive and behavioral measures (the latter consisting of a point system of rewards that could lead to increasing privileges) had no appreciable effect. Emily left the hospital after 8 months essentially unchanged. Thirteen years later at follow-up, however, I learned from her that shortly after leaving the hospital, she began treatment with a psychiatrist who prescribed a monoamine oxidase inhibitor (phenelzine). This medication had a marked calming effect and also elevated her mood. Her trichotillomania disappeared, such that she now has a luxuriant growth of hair. She was able to work, and became more amenable to the supportive interventions of her therapist, who helped her iron out her difficulties in close relationships with men. Her therapist helped her to understand that not all men were as intimidating as her father had been, nor was it necessary for her to continue her paranoid stance, viewing most others, especially men, as the "enemy." Currently, she is married, working full-time, and is asymptomatic. The phenelzine has been maintained because it seems to work well.

## Mixture of Severe Impulsive and Compulsive Tendencies, Including Pyromania

Adopted shortly after birth, a man, now 41 years old, was raised in a conventional, nonabusive middle-class family. Schizoid in personality, he grew up unable to "connect" with his age-mates or to develop friends. He became very attached to his adoptive mother. When she died of cancer during his adolescence, his behavior deteriorated. Never having been in trouble before, he then began to set fires. A compulsive diarist, he kept meticulous records of the fires he had set, which numbered 1,488 in all. In addition to this pyromania, he tortured cats and other small animals. Particularly ill at ease with women, he never dated. Shortly after graduating from high school, he was inducted into the Army and did a tour in Vietnam. There he used LSD, whereas earlier he had abused neither alcohol nor illicit drugs. He became increasingly paranoid and developed a venomous hatred of his biological mother for having given him away. Not long after his return from Vietnam he embarked on a series of murders, consisting of shooting women (and sometimes their boyfriends) who had been in parked cars along various "lovers' lanes" in New York City. The motive ostensibly was to exact revenge against "loose" women like his birth mother. Apart from this, there was no sexual element; he never committed rape or any other sexual offense. The murders took place in 1976–1977, in the course of which he mailed several letters to the authorities, the content of which was suggestive of psychosis. Long after he was apprehended and sentenced, he admitted that he had faked insanity to end up in a forensic psychiatric unit (which he viewed as comparatively comfortable) rather than in an ordinary prison.[1]

---

[1] Many will recognize this vignette as the celebrated "Son of Sam" case, in which the killer, David Berkowitz, terrorized New York City for just over a year. The details of his compulsively impulsive pyromania and, later, serial homicide are set forth in a book by Ressler and Shachtman (1992).

## Kleptomania

Debbie, a schizotypal 24-year-old woman, sought treatment for a depression precipitated by a strained relationship with her boyfriend. She lived at home with her markedly paranoid and verbally abusive father, which further added to her difficulties. Periodically she would pilfer small items from candy or grocery stores and would mention during the next therapy session that she had done so. Besides urging her not to continue doing this, I tried to "get behind" the behavior, looking at it as a symptom of some conflict or deficit in her life. There seemed to be some connection between her shoplifting—of items for which she had no use and that she usually threw away—and her chronic dissatisfaction with her mother, a meek and ineffectual woman totally subjected by the father and unable to stand up to him when he was being unfair to their daughter. But exploring this area and pointing to her feelings of deprivation—as a probable dynamic factor—did not bring her shoplifting to a halt. Matters grew worse when Debbie's father, who had been helping her with the expense of therapy, made her pay my bill herself. She now began to steal from a department store sweaters equal in value to her therapy bill. When I insisted she return the merchandise, she refused. After she did the same thing the following month and could see nothing wrong in what she had done, I told her I could no longer work with her, and therapy was discontinued.

A schizotypal 40-year-old woman had been in treatment with me for 2 years, when she began to realize that her marriage was unsalvageable. As the divorce became finalized, she grew depressed and apprehensive over being alone, and her depression was compounded by worries that she would never meet another man. One day she came to the office with a box from a department store (the same store as had been involved in the preceding case example), which she opened, tearfully admitting to me that it contained a sweater that she had walked away with but had not paid for. She had never done anything like that before in her life. She told me,

"I guess I'd better bring it back to the store." I agreed with her and asked her to share with me what may have prompted her to do this uncharacteristic act. This led to discussion of how the loneliness after her divorce reawakened similar feelings from her earlier years—of intense loneliness and deprivation, brought about by the aridity of the home atmosphere and, especially, by the coldness and exploitativeness of her mother. This woman, who was, in contrast to the preceding patient, of solid moral character, felt immense relief, the burden of guilt having been removed from her when she returned the sweater the next day.

I have maintained contact with this patient over the ensuing 20 years, during which time she remarried, much more happily this time, and continued her work as a pianist/accompanist. She has never again stolen anything. The therapy was probably helpful in her being able to select a better marriage partner, but it cannot be said to have "corrected" the "kleptomania"—of which there was but the one episode—in a woman not ordinarily vulnerable to impulsive behavior.

❖

Sharon, a woman with borderline personality disorder, manic depression, and bulimia, had already been in exploratory therapy with two different psychiatrists, for 3 years each, when moving to a different city necessitated still another change of therapist. She was 27 years old when I began working with her. Bouts of bulimia were confined almost exclusively to the 3 or 4 days before her period. She maintained normal weight by vomiting, but experienced such shame over the eating disorder and induced vomiting that the depression would suddenly intensify, sometimes to the point that she would carry out serious suicidal acts (walking in front of cars; taking overdosages of prescribed antidepressants). During these binge episodes, she would frequently pilfer inexpensive items, such as stockings, pencils, and candy bars, from stores. Immediately afterward, she would become guilt-ridden and self-denigrating—emotions that also played into the vicious circle of depression–symptomatic acts–shame/guilt–depression. She also had a number of obsessive-compulsive symptoms, most important of which was an erotomanic preoccupation with whomever she worked with in treatment.

In her thrice-weekly sessions of supportive/exploratory therapy she dwelt mostly on two themes: her father's alternating criticalness and jealous attachment to her, and her mother's generally nurturing disposition, punctuated by long periods of neglect, during which she seemed to bestow her attention exclusively on her husband. The patient became clingingly dependent on her mother, at the same time that she felt herself the victim of her mother's indifference. This latter mind-set, in which she saw herself as a motherless waif, seemed most readily connected to her compulsive (in the sense of repetitive) shoplifting, but also seemed connected to her obsessive preoccupation with her therapist. Though eager to marry and have children, she had gone several years without dating, out of fear that her father would disapprove, perhaps violently, of any boyfriend, no matter how suitable.

Medications, consisting of fluoxetine, carbamazepine, and pimozide, helped alleviate her depression and diminish somewhat the intensity of her erotomania. But no amount of interpretive work, dream analysis, or supportive measures made any real inroads in this preoccupation. The only thing that seemed promising in this regard was to restore her natural entitlements to a mate of her own, by helping her overcome her fears of her father. This work required some 2 years, but when she finally met, and became close with, a suitable man, all her symptoms—depression, bulimia, erotomania, kleptomania—quickly subsided. None reappeared over the next 3 years, apart from two brief episodes of mild depression, when the solidity of the relationship with her boyfriend was temporarily in question.

## Obsessive-Compulsive Disorder, Complicated by Intermittent Explosive Disorder

Burton, a 47-year-old lawyer, had been divorced for 6 years when he sought treatment for difficulty in establishing a new relationship. He had had a brief, passionate love affair a few years earlier, but when the woman unexpectedly left him, he went into a tailspin. Suicidal for a time, he also began to develop disabling compulsive symptoms. Always a "collector," he now amassed long-playing records and cutouts from newspapers and magazines of any and all pictures of his favorite movie stars. These items filled cartons and boxes heaped up everywhere in his small apartment, such that he could barely navigate around them. He never dared invite anyone over—assuming they could even find sitting space—lest they be appalled at the mess. In addition, he hoarded chocolates and junk food of every description, sometimes coming late for work as he detoured to take advantage of an advertised "bargain" at some grocery store.

At work, few colleagues were aware of Burton's collecting mania, but all were aware of his extreme touchiness and irascibility. During acrimonious disputes over some legal issue, he "lost his cool" on two occasions and punched another member of the firm. These episodes were preceded by a kind of prodrome in which he would "glaze over," feeling himself transported back into the time of his abusive childhood. He sometimes alienated friends with explosive outbursts of this sort and had ruined a few otherwise promising love relationships with his violent temper.

Psychologically astute, Burton had considerable intellectual insight—realizing that his temper may have come from, and had certainly been aggravated by, his equally volatile father (who had also brutalized him physically). Similarly, he could link his hoarding to his mother's habit of withholding food from him, apart from the most meager rations, out of a bizarre concern that he become "fat."

Burton's symptoms were much more powerful than his insight: they persisted in the face of exploratory therapy, supportive therapy, and even a course of behavior modification he had undergone with a previous therapist. He also had been prescribed nearly everything in the psychiatric pharmacopoeia, either without effect or with ill effect. He did not tolerate any of the newer generation of serotonergic medications, all of which either gave him severe headaches or interfered grossly with sexual function.

As for my work with Burton, there was little left to try that had not been tried before, without success, by my predecessors. Though I worked with his dreams extensively, mostly to help me get a more vivid picture of his early background, I relied, from a *therapeutic* standpoint, on very practical measures designed to curb his temper outbursts. He felt plagued by his hoarding—the effects of which he had to live with every day—yet his irascibility, though it erupted only periodically, was clearly the weak link in the chain, because it threatened his job and hence his survival. We found that small doses of thioridazine helped take the edge off his anger and his anxiety when he felt particularly "pent up." If he found himself getting into a quarrel at work, I urged him to call me at any time, at the first sign of mounting anger, before he did or said something he would regret. On two or three occasions he did get through to me during such episodes, and the attacks were aborted. After a time, just knowing I was available eased his sense of isolation. Feeling he had an ally helped him control his temper, in such a way that emergencies seldom arose.

Burton's compulsive symptoms proved more resistant. If I suggested he try to "whiteknuckle it" and *not* buy the bargain chocolates, his anxiety rose to incapacitating levels. A partial solution was eventually achieved. He managed through various excesses of thriftiness to purchase a bigger apartment. One room in the new place was now given over to the hoarded objects, and he could fill this room to the very ceiling. But he mustered enough self-control not to pile things up in the other rooms. As a result, he felt better about himself, could have company over and entertain like other people, and, while still hoarding, no longer saw himself as a hopeless eccentric. As of this writing, he is no longer in treatment, but lives more comfortably with his compulsive symptoms and is in much better control of his anger.

## Social Anxiety, Obsessive-Compulsive Disorder, and Intermittent Explosive Disorder

Thomas, 19 years of age, was hospitalized because of suicidal and aggressive acts. Schizoid in temperament, he was extremely anxious in social situations, often having been bullied and scapegoated throughout his school years by other students, both boys and girls. He was actually considered autistic during his preschool years, when he was noted to be isolated and withdrawn and constantly to rock or bang his head.

Thomas had no friends and had had no sexual experience. His parents, who divorced when he was 17, were both markedly self-centered. They were hypercritical of Thomas, the mother mocking him by saying, "I have a life and you don't." His father, whose inveterate philandering had precipitated the divorce, would goad his son to "be a man" and "get laid," even going so far as to promise to fix Thomas up with a teenage girl who was "hot for sex." But the father then humiliated Thomas by having sex with her himself in an adjoining room.

Having been torn between suicidal and homicidal feelings since about age 12, Thomas ran away from home on several occasions, took overdoses of pills at 16 and again at 18, and often "blew up" when teased by schoolmates. Though Thomas was filled with fantasies of killing his tormentors, his aggressive acts were usually limited to smashing walls with his fists. He once put his fists through a glass wall, receiving serious cuts. When he was 8, he killed a pet hamster and later tortured a neighbor's cat.

On the hospital unit he interacted at first with no one, though the other patients, especially the women, experienced him as menacing. They were uncomfortable to be around him and began to taunt him, calling him "Jeffrey," alluding to the notorious serial killer Jeffrey Dahmer, who had at that time recently been apprehended. Thomas said Dahmer's deeds "disgusted" him, yet he admitted harboring similar fantasies—of killing and dismembering people—directed mostly at women.

Thomas's stay on the unit lasted 2 years, during which time he received clomipramine and occasional anxiolytics. Twice-weekly supportive/exploratory therapy was maintained throughout his stay, as were group therapy and periodic meetings with either parent. Progress was gradual but steady. He was able to form friendships with a few of the other patients by the time he was discharged. He was less dominated by scenes of sadism and mayhem. He had come to realize that not everyone was poised to humiliate or take advantage of him, as he had originally assumed.

In the 3 years after his discharge, he lived for a while in a half-way house and he worked part-time managing a store and enrolled in college. He did not yet date women but had a few male friends with whom he would have dinner or go to a movie. His anger level was much lower, and there were no explosive outbursts. There is, of course, no way of knowing whether without the long and intensive therapy, he would have gone on to commit sadistic sexual acts. Many of the elements in the serial killer "profile" (Ressler et al. 1988) were present in his early background: sexual humiliation, suppressed rage, cruelty to animals, schizoid personality features, and so forth. We cannot as yet be completely sure that he will live the rest of his life peaceably. But Thomas has never been in trouble with the law, and the outcome thus far is encouraging.

❖

Stanley, a single 27-year-old, entered therapy because of obsessive preoccupation with a former girlfriend, with whom he had had a "hopeless" love affair 2 years before (hopeless, in the sense that she came from a different culture and her whereabouts were unknown). Living with his elderly parents, he helped out around the house but had worked only sporadically since leaving college. In personality he exhibited traits from all of the anxious cluster disorders of DSM-III-R (American Psychiatric Association 1987). Depending on circumstances, sometimes the passive-aggressive ("negativistic") component was uppermost, sometimes the avoidant. His self-esteem was low, and he suffered from marked social anxiety. He was tongue-tied when trying to ask a woman for a date; when he took a course at school, he was too nervous to ask the teacher a question.

The most prominent features of his early background, of which his memory was spotty, were a tyrannical and verbally abusive, critical father and a mother who was at first indulgent and later guilt-provoking via whiney demands and hurt expressions.

Severe onychophagia, going back to his earliest years, was his only compulsive symptom. On the obsessional side, besides thoughts about the former lover, there were intrusive and disturbing mental images, especially during masturbation, of being enslaved by, then making love to, and finally eviscerating or stabbing to death older women. He had never harmed animals or any person, with the exception of his mother, whom he struck on half a dozen occasions during the time he was in therapy. His attitude toward her, and toward his explosive outbursts, was ambivalent; he felt remorseful, and yet he also felt that he was "no kind of man" if he took her criticisms without a response.

The therapy, which consisted at first of four analytic sessions a week, was slow getting started because of Stanley's mistrust of psychiatry, which he conceived of as a kind of slick charlatanry. A therapeutic alliance was eventually established, at which point it became possible for me both to insist that he control himself whenever he felt the urge to strike out at his mother and to get him to realize that the passionately loved and hated woman of his fantasies clearly was a "stand-in" for his mother. We had to rely on psychotherapy to combat these obsessive symptoms, because he did not tolerate any of the serotonergic antidepressants. He did tolerate phenelzine, which helped significantly with his social anxiety. After a year's work on the conflicts surrounding his mother, his fantasy life grew less morbid, and he became more accepting of the more annoying aspects of his mother's personality. When she became petulant, he no longer "blew his top" and he much more easily contained his impulses to hit her.

## Severe Obsessive-Compulsive Disorder With Occasional Impulsive, Self-Destructive Behavior

Martha, a single 33-year-old, had been in treatment continuously since the age of 17, when she became agoraphobic shortly before she was to graduate from high school. The onset of agoraphobia was soon followed by the onset of crippling compulsions concerning dirt. She was unable to wear any article of clothing two consecutive days, including overcoats; anything she wore, and all her bedding, had to be sent to the launderers or cleaners the next day. Her cleaning bills were correspondingly enormous. If her parents, who paid these bills, protested, she threatened suicide, and, indeed, she had been hospitalized for self-mutilative and suicidal behavior on several previous occasions. Though she professed wanting nothing more in her life than a husband and children, she was morbidly afraid of sex, harboring frankly psychotic ideas about sperm, as though they could leap out of a man whom she merely danced with or sat next to, land on her clothing, and then make their way to her body, where they would impregnate her.

Although highly intelligent and college educated, she was never able to work, and only a year before my work with her began was she able to separate from her mother, who herself was intensely "phobic" and unable to sleep unless someone else was in the house. Martha grew up in a wealthy and highly formal home; her mother was punitive to the point of cruelty unless her daughter conformed to the rules of the house. Her mother would strap her to a chair and whip her with a belt if she suspected that Martha had "touched herself "sexually.

Therapy sessions were held four times weekly the first year and twice weekly the second. Supportive measures figured most prominently at first, because Martha was almost always "in crisis." During the brief stretches when she was calmer, some exploratory work could be done. The latter was helpful, in that she revealed for the first time to anyone the abuse history. Though she never entirely gave up the delusionary notions about sexual products, she could at least accept that her dirt phobia was, in essence, a sex phobia and that her mother was no longer likely to punish her for having a sexual life, now that she was an adult and no longer under her mother's total control. Armed with these reassurances and interpretations, Martha developed a closer relationship with a man than she had ever had before. After some months she had intercourse for the first time in her life, which she found immensely gratifying, even though she still felt compelled to send the sheets and pillowcases to the cleaners right afterward.

With respect to the dirt avoidance, she experienced some benefit from fluoxetine, but only to the point at which she could resist cleaning an overcoat for two or three days instead of one. She still had to clean paper money with detergents and had to go through complicated cleaning rituals before she could hazard eating a piece of fruit.

Because the gains she made interpersonally were not matched by similar progress in her compulsive symptoms, the decision was made, after 2 years, for her to undergo behavior modification therapy (in which the "flooding" technique was emphasized) with a specialist in this modality.

## "Pure Type" Obsessive-Compulsive Disorder

Gwen is a divorced woman, a professor of history at a local college, whom I have worked with for many years in thrice-weekly therapy. Throughout the 25 years she has lived on her own, she has never been able to leave her apartment without checking the lock somewhere between 30 and 40 times before she feels it is "truly" secured and that she can safely go on to her classes. Although her life seemed at times like a sequence of odd rituals and mannerisms, the key turning was the only one she experienced as a problem. Even so, I did not hear about that "problem" for several years, because it was actually the least of her difficulties in living. In personality, she was irritable, paranoid, and schizotypal; she had great trouble resonating with other people empathically (or, as she once put it, "I really don't grasp what makes other people tick") and tended to alienate colleagues and boyfriends with her querulousness and strange habits.

The style of therapy shifted from a mostly exploratory one in the beginning to, in recent years, a predominantly cognitive-behavioral approach. As is so often necessary with schizotypal patients, a good deal of what might be called social skills training went on during our sessions. I would take the part of some friend or shopkeeper or colleague with whom she was having difficulty, and try to give pointers on what was going wrong, how she might have interacted in a smoother way, and so forth. When, on occasion, I would focus on the key turning, she would become impatient, as though that was only a minor irritant anyway and, to her way of thinking, "incurable."

We once embarked on a program where she was to keep meticulous track of how many times she checked the lock and then to try each succeeding day to check it one time less often—as if the problem could be made to disappear in this fashion over a month or two. The experiment was a dismal failure and was abandoned after a few days. She had some intellectual insight about the symptom: she related it to the pattern her mother had established—that of locking her outside the house, tied by a leash, when company visited or when her mother did not want to be "bothered." But this insight, although probably correct, afforded her no relief.

Gwen was so mistrustful of the medical profession in general, and so paranoid about drugs in particular, that she refused even to hear my recommendations, now that the serotonergic drugs had come on the market, that she try one to see whether it could help her control her compulsive symptoms. She has benefited in a slow, incremental way from the psychotherapy, especially in the realm of relationships with men and friendships. She can maintain much longer and more satisfying relationships than was possible at the beginning of therapy. But her adamant stand against medication has left her compulsive key-turning symptom in its pristine state.

Claude, a 30-year-old single man from Haiti, had emigrated to the United States for the express purpose of finding a psychiatrist who might be able to help him with his crippling obsessive-compulsive symptoms. On the compulsive side, he had developed an overwhelming dread of stepping in dog feces when he would walk along the street. This dread led to his constantly gazing at the sidewalk and moving very slowly and defensively, such that passersby marked him as an "odd" person. On the obsessive side, whenever he would be attempting to have sex with his fiancée, the image of the Virgin Mary would suddenly appear in his mind's eye, making him lose his erection (on the assumption that She would heartily disapprove of his intended activity). This man's care was entrusted to me simply because I spoke French, even though at the time (27 years ago and long before Prozac became available) I was only a second-year resident in psychiatry.

We met twice a week. The therapy was analytically oriented, with much attention to his dreams. Claude came from a well-to-do family. His father had died many years before, leaving him to be raised by a prudish and hypercritical mother, who was strict to the letter about religion. His fiancée came from the same social stratum, but she had been divorced, and this was completely unacceptable to his mother. Claude's compulsive and obsessive symptoms developed, in fact, shortly after his mother refused to give her blessing to the union, referring to the proposed marriage as "scandalous" and to the fiancée as "disgusting."

Initially, Claude was unaware of any negative attitudes toward his mother, whom he portrayed in saintly terms. Nor did he see for a long time the connection between his fear of dog feces and the label of "disgusting" his mother attached to the fiancee. The turning point in his treatment was heralded by a dream, in which he was in a room with his fiancée, when his mother stormed in, hurling at him a roll of quite-used toilet paper. Now the connection was transparent. He could also understand that in reality his mother was being hostile and unreasonable: the fiancée was perfectly acceptable, and he had done nothing "disgusting" (and nothing offensive to the Virgin Mary) in choosing her. He felt vindicated about his choice of marriage partner and more self-confident with her during sex. His fear of dog feces subsided. The intrusive image of the Virgin came less frequently, and when it did appear, he no longer felt ashamed and frightened: he found that he could smile and wave to Her, as it were, and go on about the business of lovemaking. This successful result—the only one I have ever effected in a case of OCD through psychotherapy alone—occurred after about 5 months of treatment. A fuller description of the case was reported in an earlier paper (Stone 1970).

# Discussion

## Various Forms of Psychotherapy

Patients with what we now call obsessive-compulsive disorder were described by Pinel (1799) and LeGrand du Saulle (1875). Similar cases were known in the Middle Ages. As Baer and Minichiello (1990) note, Janet wrote about such patients at the turn of the century (Janet and Raymond 1903) and recommended forced exposure to the dreaded object in the case of certain phobias and in cases of compulsive avoidance of feared objects. The growing popularity of Freud's psychoanalytic method soon overshadowed Janet's approach, which was not revived until Marks, half a century later, advocated exposure therapy as a specific form of behavioral treatment (Baer and Minichiello 1990).

Psychoanalysts labored in the hope that understanding the meaning of the rituals or obsessional concerns would dissolve the symptoms; the notion of working directly on the disturbing rituals was, until Mark's work, deemphasized (Baer and Minichiello 1990). Analysts in the pioneering generation devoted much attention to unearthing the hidden meaning of their patients' rituals and obsessions. Abraham (1920/1948), for example, spoke of kleptomania as "often traceable to the fact that a child feels injured or neglected in respect of proofs of love" (p. 355). By taking things unlawfully, the person with kleptomania "procures a substitute pleasure . . . and at the same time takes revenge on those who have caused the supposed injustice" (p. 355).

Compulsive hand washing was described often in the early analytic literature and was almost invariably understood as engendered by guilt over masturbation (Ferenczi 1923; Goldman 1938). This assumption can no longer be considered universally applicable. I recently treated a 21-year-old college student who washed his hands 50 to 100 times a day. Extremely inhibited and reluctant to talk about his personal life, he gave no hint about the underlying dynamic during the first 2 years of analysis. When his secret was revealed, it concerned not masturbation, but, rather, that he had gotten his girlfriend pregnant when they were both 18 and had paid for her to have an abortion. Reared in a punitive and religious superstrict home, he would have been ostracized had this fact been openly acknowledged. After the revelation, the compulsion became less intense—he could shake hands with people and washed perhaps 5 or 10 times a day—but did not altogether disappear.

Now, it has become clear that compulsive rituals, whether of cleaning or of checking, although some underlying psychodynamic can eventually be discerned, can seldom be treated successfully merely by the discovery and interpretation of the relevant dynamic. Cases like Claude's, discussed in the previous section, are the exception, not the rule. Currently, cognitive-behavioral approaches will more often be employed (cf. Beck et al. 1985) and will probably prove more readily effective in symptom amelioration. As with the patients in the clinical illustrations in the previous section, there will usually be some residual problems in interpersonal relationships that may require additional supportive or exploratory interventions. Here, the choices will be dictated partly by the cognitive style of the patient and the training or orientation of the therapist. There is now substantial agreement that in the treatment of the more severe forms of OCD, combined pharmacotherapy and psychotherapy is preferable to either modality alone (Baer and Minichiello 1990). Baer and Minichiello (1990) make the further point that, in general, with OCD, "cleaners" are easier to treat than "checkers" (partly because stove or lock checking is so often done in secret and is less amenable to "flooding" that can be carried out in the therapist's office). Individuals with pure obsessions may be even more difficult to treat: "thought stopping" and other distractive techniques tend to be less effective than exposure and flooding for compulsions.

Data about the moderately long-term (2–5 years) outcome of behavior therapy for OCD have been outlined by O'Sullivan and Marks (1990). The presence of an abnormal personality exerts a negative impact on the efficacy of therapy for OCD (Rachman and Hodgson 1980), as does the presence of psychosis (Solyom et al. 1985). The case of Martha (see previous section), the patient who sent her clothes daily to the cleaners, exemplifies this last point.

General guidelines for behavior therapy of OCD, including the technique of gradual desensitization, can be found in the monographs of Wolpe (1969) and Yates (1970). Newer methods, applicable also to variants such as sexual compulsions, have been described by Josephson and Brondolo (1993) and Mavissakalian and colleagues (1985).

## Impulse Disorders and the Limitations of Psychotherapy

The impulse-control disorders named and described in DSM-IV, with the exception of trichotillomania, pose serious social problems: in legal terms, kleptomania may lead to charges of misdemeanor; pyromania and intermittent explosive disorder, to charges of felony (if, in the case of intermittent explosive disorder, serious assault and battery occur). Pathological gambling often brings ruin to the gambler and his or her family. As for trichotillomania, this condition has much more in common with a compulsive than with an impulsive disorder, because the activity tends to be repetitive and frequent, as with other behavioral manifestations of OCD. One might more properly view trichotillomania as a subtype of compulsive disorders, along with cleaning and checking. But the other four DSM-IV impulse-control disorders are often found in conjunction with antisocial personality (either with antisocial personality traits or with the full-fledged disorder), in which case the amenability to psychotherapy may be seriously reduced or nullified. This was the situation with Debbie, the patient with kleptomania and schizotypal personality disorder, and with Joseph, the patient with intermittent explosive disorder, whose cases were described in the previous section.

There seems to be tacit agreement about the reduced amenability to psychotherapy in persons with both impulse-control disorders and antisocial personality even in the earlier psychoanalytic literature, where far more space was devoted to classification and description than to suggestions for therapy. For example, Wilhelm Reich (1925), in his treatise on the "impulse-ridden character," noted that the nonorganic cases needed to be distinguished from the organic and that the nonorganic cases could be further broken down into the psychopathic/antisocial cases versus those cases representing impulsive "acting out" of the transference. In a similar vein, Frosch (1977; Frosch and Wortis 1954) focused on taxonomy of impulse disorder, suggesting a division into *symptom* and *character* varieties of this disorder, the former including intermittent explosive disorder and kleptomania. The symptom impulse disorder might have an organic underpinning such as temporal lobe epilepsy. Provided there was a pharmacological or other remedy for the organic condition, the prognosis was considered (accurately so) more favorable than when antisociality was present. Patients in whom intermittent explosive disorder develops out of some neurological condition and whose premorbid personality was nonaggressive and socially conventional are often appalled at the radical changes in their behavior, in such a way as to make them eager to comply with a regimen emphasizing medications that might minimize the tendency toward explosive outbursts. These patients will probably be more cooperative with the supportive psychotherapy that would usually accompany the medical regimen. Antisociality, in contrast, usually spells noncompliance and thus a worse prognosis. Even a markedly *externalizing* (let alone *paranoid*) cast to the personality, in the absence of distinct antisocial traits, may scuttle attempts at psychotherapy (as in the case of Beatrice, discussed in the previous section), because of the patient's failure to take responsibility for, or even to recognize the nature of, his or her behavior. If explosive outbursts occur only infrequently, there is the added problem that the patient can more easily deny that there is a problem, each incident seeming, in the eyes of the patient, to have contained such "irresistible" provocation, as though "anyone" would have lost his temper under the circumstances.

Although a few psychoanalysts continue to express optimism about the efficacy of supportive and analytic therapies in the domain of impulse disorders (e.g., Aronson 1989), the consensus now is that such claims cannot really be substantiated, apart, perhaps, from the positive results that can be achieved with these techniques in milder instances of "acting out" in patients free of antisocial tendencies. As Kavoussi and Coccaro (1993) noted, when "impulse disorder" is confined to impulsive acts of self-mutilation or suicidal gestures, as in patients with borderline personality disorder, recently developed cognitive-behavioral techniques have proven useful (Linehan 1993). For the more serious of the DSM-IV impulse-control disorders, however, when positive results are obtained at all, they will usually follow from the use of the modern mood-regulating and serotonergic drugs. A variety of 12-step programs, based on the model of AA, have also come into existence in recent years, to help individuals cope with some of the impulse disorders. Gamblers Anonymous is an example, and Sexaholics Anonymous is another. Both programs amount to a type of limit-setting, restructuring group therapy, and in this way differ from, though utilizing some of the techniques of, individual (supportive-type) psychotherapy. It is rare, in any case, for compulsive gamblers (to say nothing of pyromanic and kleptomanic individuals) to present themselves voluntarily for individual therapy.

As for kleptomania, I am not aware of any 12-step or other therapeutic programs that are considered helpful. Arguably, the most well-known example of the condition in America was the 1940s actress Hedy Lamarr—who was as famous for her shoplifting as for her beauty. Her kleptomania was not exactly cured—although it was at least rendered no longer bothersome—by the device of having herself accompanied on her trips to department stores by a private secretary whose job it was to pay the store manager on the quiet, whatever sum was needed to equal the cost of the pilfered goods. It is not known whether Miss Lamarr was fighting demons from the past, out of some troubled childhood, that had led to this symptom disorder. If not, then hers might have been a "pure" kleptomania, as that in DSM-IV, with no underlying anger or revenge motif. I suspect, though, that the same such motifs lay behind her kleptomania as are operative in less-celebrated instances.

At the crossroads between compulsive and impulsive disorders are the paraphilias, including voyeurism, exhibitionism, fetishism, frotteurism, and sexual masochism or sadism (Anthony and Hollander 1993). Placed under a separate heading in DSM-IV, these conditions partake of both repetitiveness (hence the compulsive component) and, in many instances, sudden irrepressible urge (the impulsive component). It would take us too far afield to discuss in detail the role of psychotherapy in this large and heterogeneous domain. Suffice it to say that the more chronic the paraphilic behavior and the more antisocial its nature—as in the case of repetitive sexual sadism or pedophilia—the less amenable the condition to exploratory, or even to behavior modification, approaches. Psychotherapy does have a place in the remediation of the less chronic and less socially disturbing paraphilias. As an example: A man who practiced frotteurism while riding subways, and who was successfully treated by psychoanalysis, was the subject of a recent article by Myers (1991). This man, a corporate executive, was highly motivated for treatment and was eager to preserve his marriage (he had become physically abusive to his wife also). He had been the object of much verbal abuse from his mother when he was young, and this seemed the crucial factor in his hostility toward women. When this was unraveled and worked through, his frotteurism stopped and his relationship with his wife improved.

Exhibitionism, though it would more likely be treated currently by behavioral methods, may also at times be amenable to exploratory therapy. I had occasion many years ago to treat a 38-year-old man who had been remanded by the court to a psychiatrist after he had twice exposed himself in front of schoolgirls. He had never been in trouble otherwise. In personality, he was markedly obsessive-compulsive and schizoid. He held a responsible job checking complex machinery for flaws. Apart from infrequent relations with prostitutes, he had no contact with women. Although not very aware of it at first, he harbored enormous bitterness and hatred toward women—as came out in dreams in which women in huge numbers had been massacred and were lying about in a field. His mother had humiliated him throughout his childhood. The most searing memory of this humiliation revolved around an incident when he, at age 7, was walking with her in the street. He told her at a certain moment, "Ma, I have to pee!" Pointing to a row of parked cars, she said, "Pee between the cars, you got nothing to hide!" This was the dynamic behind his compelling need, years later, to prove that he *did* have something to hide. As he grew better able to understand that not all women stood poised to mock his manhood, he became less bitter and more willing to trust women. When I spoke with him 20 years later in a follow-up effort, he was married with three children and had changed his work, to a managerial position in a store. He was no longer bitter and reclusive.

## The Abuse Factor

As is reflected in the vignettes, a high proportion of compulsive and impulsive (and one could add paraphilic) patients had been caught up during their formative years in traumatic patterns of one kind or another—physical, sexual, or verbal abuse from parents or other important caretakers. These experiences seemed to enkindle the nervous system and to lay the groundwork for later symptom development. In my own clinical work, patients with OCD were more likely to have suffered one or multiple forms of such abuse than patients who did not exhibit OCD (Stone 1993). Further research is needed to determine whether this correlation would be borne out in other patient samples. In the meantime, it would seem important to check carefully about possible traumatic factors in the histories of patients with disorders in the impulsive-compulsive spectrum.

The point here is that childhood traumas, besides tending to engender the symptomatology examined in this chapter, also routinely deform personality development in ways that severely disrupt interpersonal relationships, especially in the sphere of intimacy. These personality aberrations may take myriad forms: hostility, bitterness, lack of self-confidence, aggressiveness, distrust, and so forth. Despite the recent advances on the psychopharmacological front, it will not be common for amelioration of the personality disorder component to occur in lockstep with the subsidence of symptoms. There will far more often be a thick residue of personality problems left over, long after the compulsive or impulsive symptoms have diminished or disappeared. It is this residue that psychotherapy is best equipped to ameliorate, and for this reason, psychotherapy, in one form or another, will always have a place in the overall approach to compulsive-impulsive patients.

# References

Abraham K: The female castration complex (1920), in Selected Papers on Psycho-Analysis. Translated by Bryan D, Strachey A. London, Hogarth Press/Institute of Psycho-Analysis, 1948, pp 338–369

American Psychiatric Association: Diagnostic and Statistical Manual of Mental Disorders, 3rd Edition, Revised. Washington, DC, American Psychiatric Association, 1987

American Psychiatric Association: Diagnostic and Statistical Manual of Mental Disorders, 4th Edition. Washington, DC, American Psychiatric Association, 1994

Anthony DT, Hollander E: Sexual compulsions, in Obsessive-Compulsive–Related Disorders. Edited by Hollander E. Washington, DC, American Psychiatric Press, 1993, pp 139–150

Aronson TA: A critical review of psychotherapeutic treatments of the borderline personality. J Nerv Ment Dis 177:511–528, 1989

Baer L, Minichiello WE: Behavior treatment for obsessive-compulsive disorder, in Handbook of Anxiety, Vol 4. Edited by Noyes R, Roth M, Burrows GD. Amsterdam, Elsevier, 1990, pp 363–387

Beck AT, Emery GD, Greenberg RL: Anxiety Disorders and Phobias: A Cognitive Perspective. New York, Basic Books, 1985

Ferenczi S: Waschzwang und Masturbation. Internationale Zeitschrift für Psychoanalyse 9:70–71, 1923

Frosch J: Disorders of impulse control. Psychiatry 40:295–314, 1977

Frosch J, Wortis SB: A contribution to the nosology of impulse disorders. Am J Psychiatry 111:132–138, 1954

Goldman G: An act of compulsive handwashing. Psychoanal Q 7:96–121, 1938

Janet P, Raymond F: Obsessions et la psychasthenie. Paris, F Alcan, 1903

Josephson SC, Brondolo E: Cognitive-behavioral approaches to obsessive-compulsive–related disorders, in Obsessive-Compulsive–Related Disorders. Edited by Hollander E. Washington, DC, American Psychiatric Press, 1993, pp 215–240

Kavoussi RJ, Coccaro EF: Impulsive personality disorders and disorders of impulse control, in Obsessive-Compulsive–Related Disorders. Edited by Hollander E. Washington, DC, American Psychiatric Press, 1993, pp 179–202

LeGrand du Saulle H: La folie du doute avec delire du toucher. Paris, Delahaye, 1875

Linehan MM: Cognitive-Behavioral Treatment of Borderline Personality Disorder. New York, Guilford, 1993

Marks IM, Hodgson R, Rachman S: Treatment of chronic obsessive-compulsive neurosis by in-vivo exposure: a two-year follow-up and issues in treatment. Br J Psychiatry 127:349–364, 1975

Mavissakalian M, Turner SM, Michelson L (eds): Obsessive-Compulsive Disorder: Psychological & Pharmacological Treatment. New York, Plenum, 1985

Myers WA: A case history of a man who made obscene telephone calls and practiced frotteurism, in Perversions & Near Perversions in Clinical Practice. Edited by Fogel GI, Myers WA. New Haven, CT, Yale University Press, 1991, pp 109–123

O'Sullivan G, Marks IM: Long-term outcome of phobic and obsessive-compulsive disorders after treatment, in Handbook of Anxiety, Vol 4. Edited by Noyes R, Roth M, Burrows GD. Amsterdam, Elsevier, 1990, pp 87–108

Pinel P: Nosographie philosophique. Paris, Maradan, 1799

Rachman SJ, Hodgson RJ: Obsessions and Compulsions. Englewood Cliffs, NJ, Prentice-Hall, 1980

Reich W: Der triebhafte Charakter. Leipzig, Internationaler psycho-analytischer Verlag, 1925

Ressler RK, Burgess AW, Douglas JE: Sexual Homocide: Patterns and Motives. New York, Macmillan, 1988

Solyom L, DiNicola VF, Phil M, et al: Is there an obsessive psychosis? Aetiological and prognostic factors of an atypical form of obsessive-compulsive neurosis. Can J Psychiatry 30:372–380, 1985

Stone MH: Cultural factors in the treatment of an obsessive hand-washer. Psychiatr Q 44:11–16, 1970

Stone MH: Abnormalities of Personality: Within and Beyond the Realm of Treatment. New York, WW Norton, 1993

Stone MH: Early traumatic factors in the lives of serial murderers. American Journal of Forensic Psychiatry 15:5–26, 1994

Wolpe J: The Practice of Behavior Therapy, 3rd Edition. New York, Penguin, 1969

Yates AJ: Behavior Therapy. New York, Wiley, 1970

# 10

## Relationship Between Impulsivity and Compulsivity: A Synthesis

Larry J. Siever, M.D.

As is evident from the chapters of this book, there is increasing interest in the relationship between impulsivity and compulsivity, which perhaps represent two poles of a common spectrum. These formulations naturally raise the question of whether, indeed, impulsivity and compulsivity should be viewed as polar opposites at the far end of a single continuum or are more properly viewed as having a number of important commonalities that define the impulsive-compulsive spectrum. Although mania and depression have been conceptualized as representing opposite extremes on a single continuum, with mania representing the "high" and depression the "low," increasing evidence suggests these two affective states share many abnormalities as well. Certainly, the decreased need for sleep, increased energy, pressured speech, expansive mood, and intrusive behavior of mania contrast with the fatigue and sleep disturbance, reduced energy, depressed mood, and social withdrawal characteristic of depression. However, it is not uncommon to see "mixed" states with irritability and mixed moods of depression and mania. Furthermore, the pathophysiologies of these two states are not entirely distinct, in that both mania and some forms of agitated depression may be marked by increases in noradrenergic metabolite concentrations, reduced adrenergic receptor responsiveness, heightened sensitivity to cholinergic challenge, and reductions in serotonergic system function. Thus, although these two states are recognizably different, they may be better conceptualized as different manifestations of an underlying affective vulnerability.

A similar model may be useful in understanding the impulsive-compulsive spectrum. All of the behaviors on the impulsive-compulsive spectrum involve an abnormal regulation of active behavior in the same way that the affective spectrum encompasses an abnormal regulation of affective state. Impulsive and compulsive behaviors have in common a sense of urgency or pressure preceding the impulsive or compulsive behaviors, a relative failure to suppress these behaviors even when they are recognized as potentially maladaptive to the individual, and an underlying theoretical relationship with aggressive urges. At a biological level, arguments for an impulsive-compulsive spectrum rest on documented serotonergic abnormalities that have been demonstrated in both impulsive and compulsive disorders and the therapeutic efficacy in both sets of disorders of selective serotonin reuptake inhibitors. This common serotonergic "link" between the two sets of disorders lends more credibility to the possibility of a continuum of impulsive-compulsive behaviors. Both common and disparate elements of impulsive and compulsive behaviors may be observed in phenomenological, psychodynamic, cognitive, biological, and pharmacotherapeutic domains, and the authors of the chapters in this book effectively highlight the issues of each of those domains.

Drs. Skodol and Oldham, in their chapter on the phenomenology, differential diagnosis, and comorbidity of impulsive-compulsive spectrum disorders (Chapter 1), systematically review the DSM-IV disorders that might be included on the impulsive-compulsive spectrum. They note the similarities and differences in the manifestation of impulsive and compulsive disorders, as well as comorbidity of these disorders with each other, that challenge the notion that these represent mutually exclusive entities. For example, although psychoactive substance use disorders can be considered indications of poor impulse control and failures to inhibit cravings to abuse harmful psychoactive substances, there is a compulsive aspect of drug taking, and psychoactive substance use disorders have high overlap with other impulsive disorders such as intermittent explosive disorder, pyromania, and kleptomania (McElroy et al. 1992). Psychoactive substance use disorders are not noted, however, to have higher comorbidity with compulsive disorders, such as obsessive-compulsive disorder (OCD) or body dysmorphic disorder. Similarly, paraphilias (i.e., deviant sexual behaviors characterized by recurrent sexual urges) also have both impulsive and compulsive aspects, as Drs. Skodol and Oldham point out. Indeed, there may be a spectrum of sexual behaviors from impulsive, promiscuous behaviors that may be gratifying but represent failures to anticipate long-term consequences, to those that appear to be driven more by motivation for anxiety reduction than sexual desire. Thus, as the authors point out, the range of sexual behaviors represented in paraphilias and their context parallel issues discussed for the wider impulsive-compulsive spectrum. In eating disorders, there are also both directly impulsive elements, such as eating binges, and obsessions about body weight and exercise. Even overeating may take on a compulsive quality in that it reduces anxiety more than it provides direct gratification. Other impulse disorders such as pathological gambling, kleptomania, or pyromania also have both impulsive and compulsive features.

As pointed out by Drs. Skodol and Oldham, compulsive disorders, including OCD, also may be characterized by apparent disinhibition, as in the case of recurrent intrusion of unwanted thoughts or behaviors. Tourette's disorder, which in some cases may show a familial relation to OCD, represents a neurological illness in which dyscontrol of motor behavior in terms of verbal outbursts or tics also has a compulsive quality, although these behaviors are considered symptoms of behavioral dyscontrol rather than overcontrol. Other compulsive disorders that can be related to OCD include hypochondriasis, body dysmorphic disorder, and trichotillomania. The last-mentioned disorder also represents a failure to resist or stop impulses, in this case to pull out one's own hair, and has both impulsive and compulsive qualities. Both borderline and antisocial personality disorders, although considered impulsive personality disorders, often include compulsive features as well. In all of these disorders, a pressure for the emergence of unwanted thoughts or behaviors is resisted with various degrees of success by the individual experiencing them. Whereas impulsive acts are considered directly pleasurable in that they satisfy, for example, sexual or aggressive needs, compulsive behaviors or obsessional thoughts are considered to be accompanied by anxiety reduction, or at least the anticipation of reduction of unbearable anxiety. This distinction, however, is often difficult to make in practice, and this difficulty may account for the fact that for many of the disorders discussed in this volume, it is difficult to clearly disentangle impulsive from compulsive aspects.

To better understand the commonalities and differences between impulsive and compulsive disorders, we must move from a purely phenomenological frame of reference to a more explanatory one. Thus, cognitive, psychoanalytic, biological, and trait theory approaches have been used in attempts to explain the paradox that impulsive and compulsive disorders have both commonalities and differences. The psychoanalytic model of impulsivity and compulsivity, summarized by Drs. Vaughan and Salzman in Chapter 7, treats both impulsive and compulsive behavior as symptomatic behavior reflecting underlying conflicts. Impulsive behaviors suggest that the inhibitory capacities of the ego cannot withstand the pressure of aggressive or sexual drives. In a relatively simple model that need not even invoke psychic conflict, relatively intense drives coupled with relatively weak ego-control mechanisms will lead to direct expression of aggressive and sexual impulses. Fairly clear-cut examples of this phenomenon might be seen in individuals with organically based cognitive impairment or retardation as well as emotional dyscontrol. However, more commonly, the trigger for the impulsive behavior may not be simply the press of a drive, but rather a painful affective state generated by intrapsychic conflict. Thus, impulsive self-mutilating behavior of a patient with border-line personality disorder may be understood both as discharge of primary aggressive drive and as reduction in pervasive underlying anxiety. It is the latter hypothesis, delineated by the authors, that makes a bridge to the psychodynamic formulation of compulsive disorders.

From the psychoanalytic perspective, the compulsive disorders are also considered a response to intrapsychic conflict and its resulting anxiety. For example, Drs. Vaughan and Salzman note that a conflict over the expression of aggression toward one's father might be accompanied by compulsive checking behavior to provide assurance that the aggressive wish does not result in real damage to the father. The distinction here is between a behavior that is not directly gratifying and is designed to reduce anxiety ("undoing") and a behavior that results in a more direct gratification of aggressive wishes (self-mutilating behavior, as in the patient with borderline personality disorder alluded to above). In practice, however, behaviors that are designed to reduce anxiety are self-reinforcing in their repetitiveness, are driven by deep-seated conflict, and tend to be considered compulsive whether or not they directly satisfy aggressive or sexual drives. Thus, as discussed by Drs. Skodol and Oldham in the chapter on differential diagnosis (see Chapter 1), there is often a compulsive component to a variety of paraphilic sexual behaviors, drug use, and even self-destructive behaviors. Given that many impulsive behaviors seen in most psychiatric settings do involve some anxiety reduction, it is clear that the conceptual distinction between impulsive and compulsive behaviors may be more theoretical than practical.

According to the psychoanalytic view then, impulsive and compulsive behaviors might be considered as constituting a continuum ranging from a) the direct gratification of sexual or aggressive drives because of inadequate ego-control mechanisms, to b) direct gratification of drives driven not only by the intensity of the drives and a weak ego but also by anxiety states resulting from psychic conflict, to, finally, c) compulsive behaviors that do not involve gratification and are inevitably driven by conflict-based anxiety.

Commonalities between impulsivity and compulsivity might be found in increased intensity of aggressive and sexual drives underlying the entire spectrum of disorders. In compulsive disorders, these drives are successfully resisted in part, resulting in behaviors that do not directly gratify the drives but that can be traced back to them. In impulse-control disorders, in contrast, the drives are less successfully resisted and thus are more directly gratified. Such a hypothesis is not inconsistent with the psychoanalytic model presented and might account for the apparently more continuous nature of the impulsive and compulsive disorders.

Dr. Perry, in his chapter on defense mechanisms in impulsive and compulsive disorders (Chapter 8), logically tests this kind of hypothesis. He hypothesized that impulsive symptoms would be more related to action-oriented defenses, which allow direct expression of impulses without regard to consequences, whereas obsessive-compulsive symptoms would be more related to defenses of isolation, undoing, displacement and reaction formation, which substantially alter the underlying wish and do not provide direct impulse satisfaction. Dr. Perry's study is commendable in that the attempt is made to actually test hypotheses related to psychodynamic models; the findings from this study provide substantial, but not complete, support for such a model. Indeed, his results suggest that action and major image-distorting defenses are related both to suicide attempts and to self-cutting behaviors, as well as to substance abuse and antisocial symptoms. Obsessional defenses were not necessarily associated with obsessive-compulsive symptoms during the follow-up period.

However, as Dr. Perry notes, the data are from a longitudinal study of severe personality disorders, including borderline, antisocial, and schizotypal personality disorders, as well as bipolar II affective disorders. The impulsive symptoms were clearly related to more primitive, action-oriented defenses, but higher-level neurotic defenses might not necessarily predict the kind of severe obsessive-compulsive symptoms seen in severe personality disorders. One might conclude that compulsive behaviors, especially severe ones, may issue from very primitive defenses, as do impulsive behaviors, but that neurotic defenses might limit both impulsive and compulsive symptoms. Thus, impulsivity and compulsivity may not differ a great deal on a continuum of higher or lower defenses as psychoanalytic theory might suggest. Rather, they might reflect differences in the character of the susceptibility to symptomatology that may need to be sought in other explanatory models.

Dr. Stein, in Chapter 4, provides such a model, one driven by cognitive science. The cognitive model differs from the psychodynamic model because it is not grounded in the structural theory of psychoanalysis, with its attention to the relationship between drives, ego, and superego. Thus, a psychoanalytic model of OCD might be based on excessive anal aggressive impulses and a harsh superego. The cognitive model that Dr. Stein presents is based on the principle of fixed action patterns or specific motor sequences. OCD might be considered to involve a relatively low threshold for the initiation of repetitive motor sequences or fixed action patterns. These patterns might be triggered to ward off future harm by an overestimation of anticipated harm or by a failure to determine whether goal completion has occurred. Indeed, cognitive distortions and deficits have been documented in OCD. These deficits might be considered as parallels to "ego weakness" in psychoanalytic models. Impulsivity may also be triggered at a lower threshold as a result of cognitive deficiencies (e.g., minimization of aversive consequences of aggressive behaviors). Thus, a cognitive approach emphasizes features of behavior disturbance that are less specifically addressed in psychodynamic models (i.e., What determines individual differences in choice of defenses? Or, alternatively put, what are the substrates for the ego weaknesses implicated in both impulsivity and compulsivity?). Models incorporating both of these elements might postulate that in individuals with relatively intense aggressive or sexual "drives" or needs, excessive anticipation of future harm as a cognitive "set" might result in compulsive symptoms, whereas minimization of future harm might result in impulsive symptoms.

The domain of psychobiology and psychopharmacology may provide useful hints as to how to synthesize these models. Drs. Hollander and Cohen provide a thoughtful model of compulsive spectrum disorders in their chapter on the psychobiology and psychopharmacology of these disorders (Chapter 6). They propose that impulsivity involves a decreased estimation of harmful consequence of one's behavior along with increased risk-seeking behavior, whereas compulsive behaviors are characterized by an increased estimation of future harm and risk aversiveness. They then argue that the serotonergic system of the central nervous system (CNS) may explain these two extremes. For example, there is some evidence that increased cerebrospinal fluid (CSF) 5-hydroxyindoleacetic acid (5-HIAA), as well as increased responsiveness to serotonergic challenge, may be associated with OCD, whereas decreased CSF concentrations of 5-HIAA and blunted responses to serotonergic challenges may be characteristic of impulsive patients. This argument is brought to the neuroanatomic sphere by the authors' proposal that the hypofrontality associated with impulsivity contrasts with the hyperfrontality of compulsivity. Finally, the authors contend that the selective serotonin reuptake inhibitors may work by enhancing presynaptic serotonin in impulsive disorders and by decreasing serotonergic receptor sensitivity in compulsive disorders. The authors' arguments are logical and compelling, although there are clearly numbers of studies whose findings are inconsistent with this view. However, for heuristic purposes, the model provides a springboard for future research.

Indeed, serotonergic system abnormalities are found in a variety of disorders. It may be that different serotonergic components are altered in compulsive and impulsive disorders. For example, CSF 5-HIAA data suggest that decreases in presynaptic availability of serotonin may characterize the severe aggressive behaviors found in criminal offenders or antisocial individuals, whereas increased responses of some serotonergic receptors postsynaptically might be related to behavioral alterations in response to *m*-chlorophenylpiperazine (m-CPP) in OCD patients. Thus, not only may there be differences in serotonergic activity—whether serotonergic activity is "high" or "low"—but different components of the system may be altered in the different disorders.

Furthermore, there may be differences in interactions with other neuromodulatory systems, such as the other monoaminergic systems—the noradrenergic and dopaminergic systems. For example, in ongoing work in our laboratory, reductions of serotonergic activity have been found in both major depressive disorder and impulsive personality disorders. In major depressive disorder, these abnormalities are accompanied by reductions in the responsiveness of adrenergic receptors, whereas in impulsive personality disorders they are accompanied by normal to increased responsiveness of the noradrenergic system (Coccaro et al. 1989; Siever and Trestman 1993). Although serotonergic system deficits have been linked to disinhibition of aggressive behaviors, the noradrenergic system is an alerting arousal system that may mediate responses to the environment. Disinhibited aggression may be more likely to lead to self-directed aggression (as in suicide attempts) when accompanied by reductions in reactivity to the environment secondary to a noradrenergic deficit than when coupled with excessive reactivity to the environment due to increased noradrenergic responsiveness, which results in fighting or other forms of other-directed aggression. OCD might be understood as an excess of serotonergic activity, in contrast to depression and impulsive personality disorders, which are associated with decreased serotonergic activity accompanied by normal or heightened reactivity of the catecholaminergic system. Thus, the nature of the serotonergic system abnormality must be understood in the context of other biological systems that may affect the expression of symptoms related to the serotonergic deficit.

A biological model may then be integrated into the other models proposed above. A serotonergic system alteration may be implicated in the regulation of aggression in relation to anticipated future punishment or harm. Diminished serotonergic activity may be associated with an incapacity to modulate aggressive behavior in the service of avoidance of future punishment, whereas excessive serotonergic activity may be associated with overinhibition of such behaviors. Other neuromodulator systems and hormone systems have been implicated in aggression, including increased testosterone (Virkunnen et al. 1994). It is not hard to imagine that someone with an excessive propensity to aggression related to increased testosterone, for example, might show very different behaviors depending on whether he or she had reduced serotonergic activity or increased serotonergic activity. In the former case, direct expressions of aggression might predominate, whereas in the latter, obsessive-compulsive symptoms might emerge. These symptoms in the latter case could be understood psychodynamically as conflicts about the expression of aggression because of excessive fear of punishment (i.e., "harsh superego"). This fear might also translate into a cognitive set of greater concern about possible future harm. In this way, one can see that the various models of impulsivity and compulsivity presented in this book may complement one another and are not necessarily mutually exclusive.

Drs. Kavoussi and Coccaro, in their chapter on biology and pharmacological treatment of the impulse-control disorders (Chapter 5), focus more on disorders of reduced serotonergic system functioning and discuss some of the recent studies by Dr. Coccaro and his collaborators that suggest that reductions in serotonergic system activity are related to aggression and that the expression of aggression may depend on other systems (e.g., the noradrenergic system), as discussed previously in this chapter. Drs. Kavoussi and Coccaro note the possibility that different serotonin receptor subsystems are involved in these disorders, as well as that there may be differences in relation to other neuromodulator systems. Finally, they point out the potentially important role of early life experiences in modulating vulnerability to rapid and intensive affective shifts in response to stress in the direction of either compulsive or impulsive symptoms.

Drs. Zanarini and Weinberg document the comorbidity of impulsive and compulsive features in borderline personality disorder (Chapter 2). They conclude that borderline psychopathology is best explained by a multifactorial model, in which the psychopathology is viewed as the end product of a complex interaction between biological predisposition, early experience, and, ultimately, subtle neurological/biochemical dysfunction that may be the consequence of either a predisposition or childhood experience. However, borderline personality disorder is much more specifically related to impulsive disorders than to compulsive disorders. The authors conclude that borderline patients may have especially unstable serotonergic systems and that, for this reason, both compulsive and impulsive behaviors may be stabilized by fluoxetine.

Dr. Cloninger integrates the obsessive-compulsive spectrum into his seven-factor model of temperament and character (Chapter 3). Clearly, harm avoidance is crucial in compulsive behavior, which he believes is also characterized by low novelty seeking, high persistence, and rarely high reward dependence. In his model, impulsive behavior is characterized by high novelty seeking, low harm avoidance, low persistence, and rarely low reward dependence. Cloninger's theory encompasses dimensions that he considers more biologically based, such as harm avoidance or novelty seeking, but also others that may be dimensions of character. The latter he bases in propositional memory systems that may be shaped environmentally in the course of character development. Thus, his model encompasses both biological and environmental determinants of character development.

While acknowledging the tremendous advances in the pharmacotherapy of the personality disorders, Dr. Stone reminds us there is still an important role for psychotherapy in these disorders (Chapter 9). He argues that although impulsive and compulsive symptoms may resolve following pharmacotherapy, enduring personality disorder traits may persist, and that these may be amenable to psychotherapeutic intervention. Indeed, it is possible that individual personality "disorders" may crystallize around compulsive or impulsive predispositions in the context of specific life experiences and thus will remain somewhat autonomous even if the compulsive or impulsive traits are muted. Dr. Stone discusses his work with a number of patients with whom he used psychodynamic therapy with insight-oriented and supportive facets in which he both addressed unconscious conflicts and dispensed practical advice when it seemed appropriate. I suspect his approach is not atypical, at least for psychodynamically oriented therapists working with patients with severe personality disorders. He cites, but does not discuss in any detail, cognitive-behavior therapy, which focuses on finding alternative strategies for handling overwhelming feelings as well as on skills training. This approach seems to be particularly helpful with parasuicidal borderline personality disorder patients.

In the end, most would acknowledge that multifactorial models must be taken into account to explain impulsive and compulsive behaviors and to formulate the treatment of patients with these behaviors. However, the remarkable convergence of different theoretical approaches in relating these disorders, and the relative consistency of findings of alterations in the serotonergic system and alterations in the anticipation of future harm, associated with both impulsive and compulsive behaviors, suggest that we may not be as far from discovering potential etiological mechanisms in the development of these behaviors as we were 20 years ago. Future studies—those designed to test more specific models of serotonergic system dysfunction; the relationship between serotonergic system dysfunction and alterations in other CNS neuromodulatory systems, which includes careful assessment of cognitive deficits and schema; evaluation of both temperamental and characterologic personality traits; and assessment of defense styles—may permit us to "cross talk" between these theoretical perspectives and hopefully will yield empirical validation of an integrated perspective on the impulsive-compulsive spectrum disorders.

# References

Coccaro EF, Siever LJ, Klar H, et al: Serotonergic studies in patients with affective and personality disorders: correlates with suicidal and impulsive aggressive behavior. Arch Gen Psychiatry 46:587–599, 1989

McElroy SL, Hudson JI, Pope HG Jr, et al: The DSM-III-R impulse control disorders not elsewhere classified: clinical characteristics and relationship to other psychiatric disorders. Am J Psychiatry 149:318–327, 1992

Siever LJ, Trestman RL: The serotonin system and aggressive personality disorders. Int Clin Psychopharmacol 8 (suppl 2):33–39, 1993

Virkkunen M, Rawlings R, Tokola R, et al: CSF biochemistries, glucose metabolism, and diurnal activity rhythms in alcoholic, violent offenders, fire setters, and healthy volunteers. Arch Gen Psychiatry 51:20–27, 1994

# Index

*Page numbers printed in **boldface** type refer to tables or figures.*

Displacement/reaction formation
defense *(continued)*
summary of association with
obsessive-compulsive
symptoms, 217, **218,** 219
Dopamine blocking agents
adverse effects of, 126
in impulse-control disorders,
126
Dopaminergic function/
dysfunction
in compulsive disorders, 148
in impulse-control disorders,
124–125, 135
Drive theory, in psychoanalytic
model, 170–171, 188
Drug therapy. *See individual
agents*; Pharmacological
therapy
Dynamic unconscious, in psychoanalytic model, 168

Eating disorders. *See also*
Anorexia nervosa; Bulimia
nervosa
assessment by TPQ, 75,
78–80, **79–80**
comorbidity with borderline
personality disorder, **41,**
42–46, 47, **48**
defense mechanisms in, 219
case example of, 219–226
Fenichel's studies of, 198
impulsive and compulsive
aspects of, 263
Ego. *See also* Superego
ability to contain impulsive
drives, 175
in compulsivity and
impulsivity, 187
object representations in
formation of, 172–173
weakness of, in impulsivity, 173

Erotomania, 242
Executive function impairment,
in compulsive disorders,
150, 151
Exhibitionism, **14,** 257–258
Explosive disorder. *See* Intermittent explosive disorder
Exposure and response prevention therapy, 153, 155, 252
Eysenck Personality Questionnaire (EPQ)
erroneous assumptions of,
62–63
KSP and TPQ vs., 67, **68,** 69

Fenfluramine
in compulsive disorders, 153
prolactin response to
in obsessive-compulsive
disorder, 133
in patients with impulsive
aggression, 122–123
Fenichel, O., 196–198
Fetishism, **14**
Fixed action patterns, as model
of compulsivity, 100
Fluoxetine. *See also* Serotonin
reuptake inhibitors
blocking of
$p$-chlorophenylalanine by,
121
in borderline personality
disorder, 53, 129
in impulse-control disorders,
130
in obsessive-compulsive
disorder, 133, 134
Fluvoxamine, 134
Free association, 169
Freud, S.
cognitivist constructs and, 103
defense mechanism studies of,
195–196

Reaction formation. *See also*
Displacement/reaction
formation defense
in eating disorders, 198
in obsessive-compulsive
persons, 181
Repression, in eating disorders, 198
Reward dependence trait
assessment by TPQ
in alcohol abuse, 83, **84–86**
in anxiety disorders, 75, **78**
in cigarette smoking and
nicotine dependence,
81, **82–83**
in eating disorders, **79**
correlation among scales of
MMPI and TPQ, 73, **74**
MPQ and TPQ, 72, **72**
TCI, Eysenck's and
Norman's models, **76**
TPQ and sensation-seeking
scales, **70**
definition of, 63
validity of, 64
Risk taking
association with defenses
case example of, 225
on follow-up, **210,** 211
at intake, 205, **206, 207,** 208
predictive relationship with
defenses, 213, **215**
Rumination
pathological, in obsessive-
compulsive disorder, 101–102
serotonergic system effects on,
102

Sadism, sexual, **14**
Schema theory
application to impulsive
aggressive behaviors, 104
in cognitive science
architectures, 98–99

Schizophrenia, impulsive and
compulsive behaviors in, 6
Scripts, aggressive behavior governed by, 104, 105, 106, 109
Self-cutting
association with defenses
case example of, 223
on follow-up, 209, **210**
at intake, 204, **205, 207,**
208
predictive relationship with
defenses, 213, **214**
Self-directed character trait
correlations among TCI,
Eysenck's and Norman's
models, **77**
in Temperament and
Character Inventory, 65,
**65**
Self-mutilation, in borderline personality disorder, 48
Self-transcendent character trait
correlations among TCI,
Eysenck's and Norman's
models, **77**
in Temperament and
Character Inventory, 65,
**65**
Sensation Seeking Scale, TPQ
vs., 69, **70–71**
Sensation-seeking trait. *See* Novelty-seeking trait
Serial sexual homicide, 232
Serotonergic agents, 128–130.
*See also* Serotonin reuptake
inhibitors
Serotonergic function/dysfunction
in borderline personality
disorder, 53, 270
in compulsive disorders, 145,
147–148, 268–270
cognitive structures and,
100, 111

measurement by CSF metabolites of serotonin, 147
response to serotonin agonists, 147
summary of, 268–270
treatment with serotonin reuptake inhibitors, 147–148
in impulsive-compulsive spectrum disorders, 132–135, 262
in impulsive disorders, 121–124
animal studies of, 121
cognitive process and, 105–106, 111
correlation with CSF 5-HIAA concentrations, 121–122
genetic basis of, 123–124
pharmacochallenge studies in, 122–123
reduced CSF 5-HIAA concentrations and, 122
summary of, 270
in major depressive disorder, 269
in obsessive-compulsive disorder, 132
in ruminative processes, 102
Serotonin. *See also* 5-Hydroxy-indoleacetic acid (5-HIAA)
inverse correlation with impulsive aggressive behavior, 121–122
neurotoxins of, 121
Serotonin platelet uptake, 123
Serotonin receptors
blocking of, by metergoline, 132
mediation of impulsive aggressive behavior by, 123

Serotonin reuptake inhibitors. *See also* Clomipramine; Fluoxetine; Sertraline
in borderline personality disorder, 53
in compulsive disorders, 147–148, 152–153, 268
algorithm for, **154**
treatment resistance to, factors in, 153
in hyperfrontality, 149
in impulse-control disorders, 129–130, 152
in obsessive-compulsive disorder, 108, 133–134, 147–148
Serotonin$_{1A}$ agonists
blunted prolactin response to, 123
in impulse-control disorders, 129–130
neuroendocrine blunting in response to, 147
Sertraline, 129
Seven-factor model of temperament and character. *See* Temperament and character models
Sexual abuse. *See* Abuse (physical and sexual)
Sexual compulsions. *See also* Paraphilias
in paraphilias, 13–15
response to serotonin reuptake inhibitors, 152
12-step programs for, 256
Sexual homicide, serial, 232
Sexual masochism, **14**
Sexual sadism, **14**
Sjobring's model of personality, 63
Smoking, assessment by TPQ, 80–81, **81–82**